GRACE
INFUSIONS

To Melanie —
So great to
meet you —
Looking forward to
more of God's
Grace in our
lives —
MB

GRACE INFUSIONS

A NURSE'S LIFE: FROM THE CRAZY TO THE HEART WRENCHING

MARYBETH SEAL

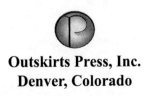

Outskirts Press, Inc.
Denver, Colorado

Grace Infusions
A Nurse's Life: From the Crazy to the Heart Wrenching
All Rights Reserved.
Copyright © 2011 MaryBeth Seal
v2.0

Cover image provided by MaryBeth Seal

Outskirts Press, Inc.
http://www.outskirtspress.com

ISBN: 978-1-4327-6884-3

Outskirts Press and the "OP" logo are trademarks belonging to Outskirts Press, Inc.

PRINTED IN THE UNITED STATES OF AMERICA

Dedication

I dedicate this book to my husband Rob, who is a
gracious man, musician, and also a nurse. Thank
you for your loving encouragement and faith in
me. To my son Benjamin, who has always been
a true grace giver and the son of my happiness.
And to my mother Margaret, the best cheer leader
any one could ever want; not only to me; but to all
seven of her children.

Contents

Introduction

I was not the little girl who always wanted to be a nurse when she grew up. The thought first entered my mind at age 16 when my high school offered a class for "hospital aides" for those students who were interested in healthcare as a vocation.

I had some interest so I signed up. After a period of classroom preparation, we made our first trip to the hospital. The only other time I really had any hospital experience was when I was in the third grade and was stricken with pneumonia so badly that I was admitted for a week to the pediatric ward.

On my first day, feeling quite pretty in my new pink hospital aide apron and shaking like a leaf inwardly, I received my orders from the nurse at the nurse's station. I was to go in room number____ and feed Mr.____. *I can do that!* Feeling confident and competent to be able to complete my assigned duty from the nurse in charge, I searched the hall to find the room and my patient.

I entered the silent room and saw an elderly black gentleman laying in a fetal position in the bed. His bedside tray had on it a liquid like farina in a bowl and a huge syringe, the size of which I'd never seen or imagined, next to it.

The man's tongue protruded snakelike in and out of his mouth rather rapidly. He didn't seem to hear me when I spoke to him and his eyes gazed up, down, and everywhere but to my voice. I had no idea what to do with the stuff on the tray, was frightened of the man in the bed, and felt totally inadequate to know to do.

With my confidence and competence between my legs like a shamed dog's tail, I left the room. I decided that day, nurse work was not for me. I couldn't get the debilitated man's face out of my mind. The pity I felt for his condition was more than I could bear, and it made me feel sick to my stomach. Thirty six years later, this man's face is still in the picture files of my mind's computer.

At age 18, I was back at the hospital on my first job as a ward clerk in the Emergency Room. I was good at typing and thus the job of checking in patients at the E.R. window. I felt adequate at this and learned a lot about general hospital lingo like "STAT", "Respiratory therapy to room__", "Code Blue", and more. The E.R. front desk was never boring and I thoroughly enjoyed the work.

After marrying and having our son, I became a stay at home mom. When our little boy was five I gravitated back to the hospital for a ward clerk job again. This time it was not in the E.R. but on a medical surgical floor. The job was the same but different. I learned more about doctors' orders, medications, medical terminology and sat in the center of the nurse hub. I got to know some of the nurses and began to think, "I could do that job." I was now 24. I also wanted to make more money! So, I signed up for nursing school at a nearby college with much encouragement from my husband who had said many times if he'd said it once, "I think you would make a good nurse."

Needless to say, nursing school to me was like a fountain of refreshing water and my brain downed the information-- like a man stranded in the Sonoran Desert on a mid July's day. I couldn't get enough fast enough!

Now, almost thirty years later, I reflect on the decision to become a nurse as a true blessing. The people I've met, the places I've gone, in the States and out of the States, have given me great experiences and memories.

Probably some of the most important things I learned were not all about the medical things like I.V. lines, tests, and medications. It was about people. Often it was about myself. Very often it was about God's grace in diverse situations with both.

I have been a nurse to the rich and the poor--to the intellectual and the mentally destitute--to white people and people of diverse color. I think I've caught a glimpse of how God views people from all walks of life. He loves because he loves. He gives us his abundant grace because he just does. He created all people in his image. As we see him as he is, we can reflect his goodness to others. Sin has devastated us, but grace has saved us.

I have a flash back of a patient of mine that was on hospice. He was an alcoholic dying of cirrhosis. I found him one morning in his bathtub with the tub water facet on full blast. He was barley hanging onto life and a belt he had strapped around the bath bar as he floated atop with his face mostly submerged. after I phoned for help; he was placed in a nursing home. Now he was dying from aspiration pneumonia.

I felt unusual compassion this man and put my

hand on his head to pray for him in his last moments. He was barely conscious yet he reached his bony arm up to push my hand away. To this day, I still wonder why. Is it possible he'd never come to realize the gracious love of God? That thought to my mind was more disturbing than finding him drowning in his own bathtub.

My hope is that you will catch a glimpse of God's grace and love as you read "Grace Infusions." God's grace is available. It is abundant. He never runs out. You don't have to feel it to believe it. It's there. Receive it. Believe it. Share it.

Grace Infusions

"The grace you had yesterday will not do for today. Grace is the overflowing favor of God; you can always reckon it is there to draw upon. In much patience, in afflictions, in necessities, in distresses, we need grace.""

Quote from My Utmost for His Highest,
Oswald Chambers.

Grace for the moment. Grace for now.

I need grace to write this book. I need grace this moment because poison ivy rash is invading my left forearm like an army of ants on a dead carcass. It's been a constant irritation during the past few days, despite steroid creams, pills, and remedies. But it is also a tool to prod me into doing that which God has called me to do. I tried to do some weeding outdoors but the warm, sticky air seemed to inflame my rash unbearably, like gas on a smoldering fire. It drove me back into the safe coolness of my house; this, too, is a grace to me. So I headed back into my office to write, as I should have been doing, instead of procrastinating on my assigned work.

I often ask God for a *grace infusion*. I need them daily, actually more than I need coffee, tea, or anything that charges my battery. As a nurse, I've helped people get infusions of all sorts. Blood, electrolytes, antibiotics, chemo drugs for cancer… just to name a few. I've seen nurses and doctors ask for "IV caffeine!" more than once at the coffee pot station.

My 86-year-old mom is going to receive an iron infusion for anemia. Her body cannot replace all of the red blood cells she lost in a recent bleeding ulcer, so she needs to be infused. Interestingly, the hematologist who will be treating her anemia told us during a specialized doctor visit: "The country of America is presently out of iron. We have a very short supply that we reserve for our sickest patients, such as those with leukemia. We won't have any for about four to six weeks. We will let you know when we have enough to treat you."

Out of iron? We'll let you know? It sounded like he was saying, "Sorry. Come back again. We are all out of help for *you* today." Though we understood the situation, our hopes were a bit dashed that she wouldn't be feeling as well as she could be with an iron transfusion. Feeling weak from anemia is not very pleasant. Feeling weak from any illness or infirmity can be distressing.

America may be out of iron. Doctors may be out of answers. We may be distressed and infirm. But God is never fresh out of grace. Never out of love and care for us. Never out of compassion or mercy. Never short on grace.

And we can get it now. No appointments needed. No needles involved. Do you wonder how?

We don't have to wait. Wise Oswald Chambers states this about grace: "It is not a question of praying and asking God to help you; it is taking the grace of God *now.* Don't say I will endure this until I can get away and pray. Pray *now;* draw on the grace of God in the moment of need. Prayer is the most practical thing, it's not the reflex action of devotion. Prayer is the last thing in which we learn to draw on God's grace." (June 26 - My Utmost for His Highest.)

I used to procrastinate in prayer for that very reason. I thought I had to *get away to pray; or be in the proper position.* Now I pray while sitting on an exam table before the doctor enters the room to see me. I pray in bed when I feel too weak to get up and do my daily work. Yesterday, with arms around my elderly mother, with tears falling down both our cheeks, I prayed for grace for my mother's loneliness and help for both of us. And days before, I prayed aloud while standing in our garage for God to help me and my husband place the decals properly on the boat he is fixing up so we can go fishing.

Grace is always available. Nothing is too big or too small to pray about. I am amazed that at the very moments when I call upon the Lord, he is hearing my lowly and seemingly unimportant requests. Though there are far more urgent issues, an almighty God in heaven, the High and Holy One, bends his ear to hear the pleas of one of his many, many children. Amazing grace from an amazing God whose goodness is unfathomable---it's available to you and me.

These words from an old hymn infused me this morning. I've never heard it sung but I poured over the print in an old hymnal of ours. I even sang it aloud. Though I am not very musically inclined; I still received an infusion!

GRACE INFUSIONS

Fill Me Now

Hover o'er me, Holy Spirit,
Bathe my trembling heart and brow
Fill me with thy hallowed presence,
Come O come and fill me now.
Thou canst fill me gracious Spirit,
Though I cannot tell thee how;
But I need Thee greatly need Thee,
Come O Come and fill me now.
I am weakness, full of weakness,
At Thy sacred feet I bow;
Blest divine, eternal Spirit,
Fill with power and fill me now.
Cleanse and comfort, bless and save me,
Bathe O bathe my heart and brow
Thou art comforting and saving,
thou are sweetly filling now.

Chorus

Fill me now, fill me now, Jesus, come and fill me now;
Fill me with Thy hallowed presence,
Come O come and fill me now.

Grace for Failures

"I am ruined, for I am a man of unclean lips…"

Is. 6:5

This Sunday our pastor was in rare form. "Do you try to force the hand of God in your life?" he declared. "Do you only obey for the blessing? Do you use God as a plan B in your life? You know, you go about your life and ask God to fill in the blanks that you've created in your own wisdom or strength."

I squirmed. I was guilty. Yes, yes and yes were my answers to his piercing questions. I don't know what anyone else answered but I knew all of my intentions to serve God were not pure, not holy or righteous. Many of them were self serving and I felt sorrowful---aghast that I, who love God, who profess to serve him, am guilty of impure motives in my relationship with him. It broke my heart.

Sins, failures, impure motives, we all have them. Sometimes I feel overwhelmed by the heaps of past failings in my life: in my marriage, in my relationships with friends and family members, in my own inability to fulfill the goals I desire.

The night before this Sunday sermon, I heard this song come to me by an invisible Messenger. *"I, the Lord of sea and sky, I have heard my people cry…I have wept for love of them…Whom shall I send?"* I knew this Messenger was none other than the Holy Spirit wooing me and speaking to my heart. I thought perhaps it was a special message about going back to Borneo for more medical missions as I've done in the past few years. I mused over the lyrics in my mind; over and over I let them roll over me like waves of the sea.

As worship began at church the next morning, our worship leader expounded on Isaiah, chapter 6, regarding the call of Isaiah. He told of the holiness of God first, where God was seated on a throne, and the seraphs covered their eyes and feet as they proclaimed the holiness of God. The temple shook and was filled with smoke.

Next he described Isaiah's reaction in verse 5 when he proclaims, "I am ruined! I am a man of

GRACE FOR FAILURES

unclean lips and I live among a people of unclean lips, and I have seen the King, the Lord Almighty!" He recognized his sinfulness and that he was not holy or pure. He had no right to be in God's presence. He had no hope either that he could ever be so—based on his own merits, strength or wisdom.

Then one of the seraphs took a live coal which he had removed from the altar and touched Isaiah's mouth and said, "See, this has touched your lips; your guilt is taken away and your sin atoned for." There was nothing magical about this coal in itself, it was God who cleansed Isaiah and forgave his sin (verse 7).

I feel undone when I see my sins, my faults, impure motives, and hear words that pass through my own lips shocking me at times. We may think to ourselves *I'd never say that* and then we do.

But as the seraph informed Isaiah that his guilt had been taken away and his sins atoned for, we too have been informed by God that his Son, Jesus, has taken our guilt away and our sins, too, have been atoned for.

Isaiah did acknowledge and confess his sins as he proclaimed, "Woe is me! I am a man of unclean lips!" We too must acknowledge and confess our wrongdoings, sinful thoughts, deeds and words.

If we confess our sins, God is just and faithful to forgive them. Now that's grace. No penance, no more guilt, but restoration with the God who radically loves us.

When I was a kid, I attended a church where I was required to do penance after a time of confession. Truth be known, I would dutifully start out saying my many prayers for my assigned penance and ultimately would lose track of how many times I'd said a prayer and would have to start all over. I found this process entirely frustrating and ended up feeling like I must be a hopeless case for God because I couldn't even do my penance right! I'd go away from the church feeling like I let God down and I would never be quite right in his sight. *Perhaps there was something just wrong with me. Everybody else could probably count their prayers just right—but not me.*

Ever felt that way? You just don't measure up? Probably never will? After all, look at how many times you've failed in the same area, over and over again. There couldn't possibly be enough grace for that---could there? There must be a point at which God has simply reached his limit with us---like we do with others such as our kids when they continually misbehave and we lose it. Does God have

GRACE FOR FAILURES

a grace limit? How much grace does he have for addicts? For abusers? For winners or losers? For liars, thieves and cowards? How much grace does God give?

Grace, grace, God's grace. Grace that will pardon and cleanse within.
Grace, grace, God's grace. Grace that is greater than ALL my sin.

His grace is enough. His shed blood once and for all, is and was enough for *all* of our sin. Today's sin, tomorrow's sin, and yesterday's too. It's enough.

Outrageous Grace

God's grace if often showcased best in the midst of our toughest trials. When we've made the worst mistake, when we've exhausted all of our own strength, and when all hope disappears from the shores of our pain and heartache, God shows up. No matter what sins have marked our past, grace is the eraser that wipes the slate clean. In the realm of God's all-powerful grace, we find His forgiveness----

DAILY GRACE, pg 19

"I will love you no matter what you do," my father cried, kneeling at my bedside at dawn one morning. Tears streamed his permanently tanned face. The only other time I'd seen him cry was at his mother's funeral. I felt as though a king was prostrate before a lowly, unworthy, unfaithful servant.

GRACE INFUSIONS

I was eighteen years young with a huge attitude. I was rebellious, deceitful, and self righteous. I would have my way no matter what. No matter that it was breaking the heart of my own father who gave his life for me and my six siblings, day in and day out laboring for a meager wage by the sweat of his brow. I was going to get married with or without his blessing. Months of screaming battles and silent wars had filled our home because of my defiance and immaturity. I was blind, like teenagers can be, not fully knowing the harm I was causing to my family, especially my parents.

One month before I did marry, my father entered my bedroom and knelt by my bed. He rarely crossed the threshold of my room. The only other times I remember him entering my room was to bring a basin when I had the stomach flu, or to prop me up in bed so I could breathe easier during bouts with asthma.

There, kneeling before me, the strongest man I'd ever known held my hand and said those words I will never forget. "I will love you no matter what you do." This was a man of action, not words. I never heard him say "I love you," to anyone including myself before this moment. He was from south Chicago. He had a physique that guys dream of—the six pack and bulging biceps were from hard work, not working out hard. He was in World War II. He was a man's man. But, on his knees before me, he was a noble king. A humble, noble king.

My father was not a religious man. As a matter of fact, most Sunday mornings he claimed that he was closer to God in his *garden* than the man behind the robes and podium. He did not go to church with us. But he was honest and real, and he did fear God. I know this because as the moment of his death from cancer neared, he called for the priest, to confess. He knew he needed to be right with God before his death. In his frailty, only days before his death, he asked to see a priest.

As a hospice nurse, I have attended many deaths. Many people don't think of confession, a priest, a pastor, or a prayer before they enter eternity. When my father asked to see the priest, I knew, at the mature age of 20, that he feared God and wanted to do the right thing before he died. This spoke volumes to me, though much of my own view of religion, Christianity and being "saved" was a blurred jumble of spiritual jargon. As I now write this at the age of 50, I know that humility and confession of sin is one of the most basic foundations of Christianity and that God hears and forgives. He who told the thief: 'Today thou shall be with me in Paradise,' forgives at the death bed as a life sputters to an end.

Grace, outrageous grace. My father extended outrageous grace to me that morning and later walked me down the aisle. We both shed tears. I adored him. His love for me has helped me see, understand, and to know God as my loving father, and I am a very blessed person for having had Alois John Vlasicak as my earthly father. I don't idolize my father. I can make a list of his many faults and sins that would be quite lengthy, but his example of humility and love toward a stray-ing, rebellious daughter left me with an example of outrageous grace that is imprinted on my heart and mind forever.

God is able to make all grace abound toward you—2 Cor. 9:8. God is able; we are not. He makes grace to be plentiful and to flourish toward us. There is nothing we can do to make God love us more than he already does—and he can never love us less either. His grace is amazing.

Remembering acts of grace in our lives is a good exercise for the soul. It reminds us of the enormity of God's love and goodness. Take some time…write your own stories down. Reflect, muse, and let *grace infuse* you. A good cup of time must be pondered and absorbed—it needs to sit and soak. We need to rest and meditate on the knowledge of God's goodness and grace and savor the flavor of his love.

Grace for Dummies

Dummy is not a nice word.

I used to feel very intimidated when I came across that striking yellow book that read *Computers for Dummies* because it revealed that I was one of them. I was computer illiterate. I-- was a dummy.

Even though I graduated from nursing school, worked some very challenging jobs and had a good mind, I was a dummy when it came to computers. The word dummy jabbed at my self esteem. It threatened to convince me that perhaps I really was and always would be one when it came to computers. Dummy is not a nice word. It means to be stupid. No one likes to be called stupid, feel stupid, or to be thought of as stupid.

As I have been reading more about God's grace

I have begun to feel like a dummy. Not because I don't understand that his grace is absolute unmerited favor---I do. I know in my heart that there is nothing I can do to make God love me more and that there is absolutely nothing I can do to make him love me less. However, I am dumb when it comes to *giving it* to others.

One of my favorite Bible passages is in the book of II Samuel, chapter 9. David had finally become king of Israel and established his kingdom. He asks "Is there anyone still left of the house of Saul to whom I can show kindness for Jonathan's sake?"

While establishing his rule, many descendants of Saul's family were wiped out. But David, being a leader of integrity, demonstrates great compassion and mercy by asking this outrageous question.

Jonathan, son of Saul, was David's dearest friend. They were kindred spirits. Saul, on the other hand was David's enemy, though David harbored no animosity toward him. Saul chose to follow his own wicked, jealous heart and sought to destroy him. He hunted him down for years like precious prey.

In spite of this, David desired to bless someone in the house of *Saul*---for Jonathan's sake. He obviously wasn't a grudge holder. Grudges have a way of invading our relationships and can extend on down the line through generations: Aunts who don't speak to their sisters or sisters in law for years; fathers and sons who carry on prideful behaviors that break down other relationships in the family, siblings who don't forgive one another, friends who don't care about one another anymore. And yet it was David's desire to bless someone in the family line of someone that *hated* him. It wasn't for Saul's sake, but Jonathan's. But it was *still* in the lineage of Saul's family.

So there was one person found. He wasn't a commander of Saul's army. He wasn't a wealthy landowner. He was a son of Jonathan's. He was a cripple. His name was Mephibosheth. He was crippled in both feet from a young age.

David tells him that now he is the new king of Israel, he will restore to him all the land that belonged to his grandfather (Saul) and that Mephibosheth will always eat at his table.

The cripple bowed down and said, "What is your servant, that you should notice a dead dog like me?"

Talk about poor self esteem! I have felt like a dummy but never a dead dog!

GRACE INFUSIONS

I can actually say I've had the experience of sitting at a king's table. Well--almost. I was a private duty nurse for an elderly woman who was a billionaire; her husband's British family lineage included royalty. The only thing they lacked was the official titles of "Queen or King."

Going to the twenty-six room mansion to nurse the lady was definitely out of my comfort zone. I did enjoy caring for this prominent elderly woman, however, and learned some interesting things about the extremely wealthy.

One of the first things I learned was that I was not one of them! My first day on the job, I was instructed to eat my lunch in the kitchen where the domestic servants ate and *not* to attend to my patient in the dining room where she ate with her husband and the butler.

The formal dining room was a completely separate room. The silver candlesticks, and tableware were cleaned on a weekly basis whether they needed it or not. In two years of taking care of this lady, I only saw the formal dining room used once at the holidays. And it was extravagantly elegant.

As my patient's condition declined, I was asked to come into the dining room where she ate with her husband. Like the Jefferson's, I felt like I was *moving on up* in the world to be sitting at the same table! I observed the butler standing by the distinguished gentleman, with a towel over his arm, pouring wine at the right time as needed. He stood like a statue for the long dinner hour (or longer, many nights).

Sitting at the table of royalty is not a little thing. So it was a great act of mercy and kindness to allow this physically deformed relative of King David's enemies to sit at the king's table on a daily basis. Huge grace again---outrageous grace.

Do you think it's possible that Mephibosheth was looked upon as a dummy by those around him? He was crippled in both feet; therefore if he could walk at all it would have been a sad sight. His gait would have been indescribably odd. I don't know what they had for wheelchairs back then; but even his transportation would probably have appeared odd to us. People who have physical handicaps are often looked upon as unintelligent. As a nurse, I have witnessed this very unfortunate attitude.

One of my most unforgettable patients was a young man with Duchene's Muscular Dystrophy. At the age of 26 he was completely wheelchair bound with no use of arms, hands, or legs. He couldn't even breathe on his own and was therefore dependent on a portable ventilator. Taking him out in public was always a challenge because of all the equipment on his wheelchair, and because of the deformities muscular dystrophy had left on his extremities. I don't know which were more humiliating to the young man: the rude stares or the intentionally averted eyes.

He was one of the smartest, kindest, and most courageous patients I've ever had the privilege of caring for. We became friends. Years later, I was proud to hear that he'd graduated from Montana State University. Our ten-year-old son learned how to play chess from him. He was certainly not a dummy. His body was broken, but not his brain or emotions.

A cripple at the king's table; think about it. You and I are cripples too. We are debilitated by sin. We are all like "dead dogs" and yet Jesus calls us to the banquet table with him. There is a seat ready there for you and me.

God graciously offers us forgiveness of sin and a place in heaven. We may feel unworthy. The truth is we are completely unworthy. Whether you are a church girl, a prostitute, a drug dealer, or a liar and a thief; we are all sinners and worthy of nothing but death and hell. Jesus gave his life, a costly gift that we can never repay.

GRACE FOR DUMMIES

Jesus said, "Here I am! I stand at the door and knock. If anyone hears my voice and opens the door, I will come in and eat with him, and he with me."

The challenge to us as believers is: will we ask others who are debilitated by sin to sit at the same table with us and Jesus? Will we ask them over to lunch at our house? Maybe serve a meal at the local rescue mission? Will we be kind to the mentally disabled or physically challenged? Will we give grace to someone who has offended us?

Grace for dummies. Don't be one. Give some.

And Grace, My Fears Relieved

God holds us in the palm of his hand...

Like a stealth bomber, it came, it dropped its load, and disappeared.

The summer skies burst open and showered a downpour of rain onto our thirsty lawn. The clouds furiously emptied their loads of moisture. Oddly, despite the raindrops pounding our deck and lawn, there was an eerie silence. It was a silent outpouring of grace in the middle of July. The dark clouds snuck in and deluged the earth below with heavenly water.

Like rain storms, dark clouds of fear are apt to sneak up on us, too, in different seasons of our live. All of a sudden they are there without warning. Dark shadows threaten our souls and cast doubts that make us anxious: the health problems that never cease, the misunderstandings and mixed messages in human communication, and the concern for our future assail us on a daily basis, not to mention sin that is ever present in our members.

I need grace in these times. When I don't know what to do, where to go, or who to call, I need grace. *Whom do I have in heaven but you, oh Lord? Who knows my way? Who cares for my soul? My soul is in a drought; bring me thy rain of grace.*

Amazing grace, how sweet the sound, that saved a wretch like me. I *once* was lost but now am found, was blind but now I see. I oft feel wretched, lost, and in the darkness. One of the amazing things about grace is that it isn't available only *once*. Not just *once* in a lifetime, not just *once* a day, but on a continual basis as needed.

My mother's one annual osteoporosis treatment is supposed to protect her; God's grace is given as needed. I used to give pain medications on a PRN basis to my patients; meaning as they *needed* it. If they were in such a state mentally or physically in which they could not ask for it, I would assess their physical symptoms, their countenance, whether they were clenching their hands or not. I would check their vital signs for duress and changes that would indicate discomfort or suffering. They didn't have to do anything special or behave in a certain manner for me to medicate them. I gave it as they needed it.

It's comforting to know that we can receive God's grace for times of fear or stress by asking for it. What is even more amazing is that, at times when we cannot ask, Jesus himself assesses our need and asks the Father for help on our behalf. He delivers comfort and relief to us as needed.

Fear is not a new problem; it continues to be an enemy that assaults the believer on a regular basis. Sometimes it's an all out battle, sometimes it's like a nagging gnat buzzing near our ears and causing a constant annoyance. Nonetheless, we need grace to relieve our fears.

The *what ifs* that plague our thoughts can back us into a corner or incapacitate us; paralyzing our ability to function in daily tasks. Grace relieves the need to know the future or the outcome. Grace says, "Everything will be all right," whether things look all right or not.

"My grace is sufficient for you," is what God told Paul regarding his affliction. "My strength is made perfect in weakness." My grace is 'adequate, plenty, or enough' are other ways to express sufficient. God's grace for our fears is adequate, plenty, and enough to deal with them. *God can make a way where there seems to be no way; he works in ways we cannot see----he will make a way for me,* so goes the song. I can't make a way, but he can. I'm not smart enough, but he is. I'm not strong enough—or brave enough…..but he is. He is at work; though I cannot see it, I believe it.

Being raised with two sisters and four brothers left me a bit people-dependent you might say. I was never alone! As I grew up and moved out on my own, I had a terrible fear of being alone. I remember feeling afraid if I were alone in the house, especially at night. It left me feeling very anxious.

Aren't we that way even as adults, though we're often not fully conscious of our behaviors and anxieties? We don't want to be alone in this world. We don't want to be abandoned or rejected. Yet in the real world that we live in, people do abandon us whether literally or emotionally. We fret and panic and forget that God himself will never leave us nor forsake us. He understands our frailty and cares for us. His eye is on the sparrow, and he is watching us.

Recently I went to our garage to paint something and saw a tiny bird on the cement floor. *It must be a baby bird* I mused, as I stooped down to inspect it.

I tenderly grasped the wee brown bird and placed it my palm. It didn't move, or peep or try to peck me. It just sat on my palm looking at me. I was tempted to find a cage for it because it was cute, and I didn't want a hawk to get it like it had my two baby chicks the year before. Instead, I went to place it in the grass under a bush in hopes that its mother would find it. Before I could set it down it lit off my hand into the bush! It was able to fly---not as helpless as I thought! What a delight it was to hold such a fragile life and also to observe its sturdiness, though so frail.

God holds us in the palm of his hand. His eye is on the sparrow. Let his grace relieve your fear.

Grace for Unquiet Minds

WANTED: Extreme Grace

Six million or more Americans have unquiet minds. Bipolar disorders afflict the rich, poor, famous, unknown---people from every walk of life.

We watched the movie titled "A Beautiful Mind" once again last evening. Russell Crowe was brilliant in this movie as he portrayed a Princeton professor with an unquiet mind. Plagued by paranoid delusions and racing thoughts, he eventually had a mental meltdown that landed him in an institutional setting for what appeared to me as a brutal form of therapy for his afflicted mind. Eventually he returned home to his wife and son and humbly tried to fit into society once again. The film portrayed the grace and 'ungrace' of society toward this eccentric professor in real ways that one could not imagine. The rejections, teasing, jeering, suspicious gazes, are scenes we have all witnessed or been party to in real life.

Perhaps even more brilliant was the part his wife played. She displayed a graceful woman who loved her man despite erratic and peculiar behaviors such as talking to people who were not there and being obsessed with solving mathematical equations for hours on end. She saw something others didn't see. She saw his heart and the man he was beyond his unquiet mind. She exhibited extreme grace.

Over the past months I have had many opportunities to talk with and work with people who have unquiet minds. When I note disjointed speech flying faster than the AM TRAC or when I wonder why they are so self absorbed, instead of thinking, "Wow, what a brain case, I realize that they constitute a few of millions afflicted with an unquiet mind and that they are not *whacked* out or possessed by a demon.

Why would I say something like that? According to an article I read recently in BIPOLAR Magazine, about one third of religious people still stereotype mental illnesses as a spiritual or sin problem. To the dismay of those who live with these afflictions, they are often rebuked by their spiritual leaders or friends for being born with unquiet minds. Heaping accusations on top of the self accusations that assault them on a daily basis is not what a person with an unquiet mind needs. They need grace.

At a recent social I attended I met friends from my youth. It had been almost thirty years since I'd seen them. We noted that our bodies had changed and aged, but we also realized that some things had not. The extraverted personalities were still outgoing, and the quirky personalities were still quirky. Those with personality problems still suffered from them. I didn't know what bipolar was as a teen, but as a nurse, having studied and treated patients with the disorder, it helped to understand and identify its cardinal symptoms.

I confess, before I understood it, I, too, was judgmental, prone to criticism, and ungracious to those who live with their particular unquietness. I was even mean and unkind in my thoughts and actions.

A Beautiful Mind portrays a true story of suffering and grace. It's on my list of top ten movies. Whether we have a mental disorder or not, there are times when we all have unquiet minds and need understanding.

Anxiety plagues millions of people too. I personally have suffered with generalized anxiety for as long as I can remember. As a small child, I would cry if I thought the gas gauge was getting too low! What's that about? My parents never ran out of gas but yet my young mind was plagued by such possibilities for no apparent reason.

When anxiety is great within me, your consolation brings me joy Psalm 94:19 . This is a verse that infuses comfort to my soul when I feel troubled and anything but quiet inwardly. Sometimes we need to sit down and hook up to the Word and let it *infuse* us. It may not feel like it's doing anything at that moment, but its effects will certainly work in time because God's word is powerful and will accomplish its work in us and will bring us peace.

Father in heaven, help me to love and understand those with unquiet minds. Let me not be of a critical spirit, but help me to be gentle and kind. Infuse me with your grace when I myself experience unrest and anxiety, and fill me with your grace for others who need your consolation.

Chosen by Grace

How great is the love the Father has lavished on us that we should be called the children of God!

I John 3:1

She lives in a four room house. I have a four car garage. She was born in Benton Harbor. I was born in Chicago. Her daddy died when she was very young. My dad died when I was twenty. She is mentally challenged, unwed, and having her fourth child. I've been married for thirty one years, have an adult son and have had a career as a nurse. I'm white. She's black. She lives one mile from me.

I have Maytag front loaders in my house. She pushes a stroller to the Laundromat stuffed with wet clothes to dry. I drive to the grocery store. She takes Dial-A-Ride. We both like perfume and perfumed soap. I like girly clothes. She likes t-shirts and jeans. She walks to Walgreen's to get her meds and to KFC for a piece of chicken. I go through the drive-through in my Mitsubishi.

I watched her get three rotted teeth pulled by a dentist who roughly kept demanding that she keep still. Then she passed out in my car on the way home. I dropped her off at the Emergency Room and asked the nurse there to help her immediately because she was pregnant. I have all my teeth at age fifty.

Why was she born to poverty, while I had parents who took good care of us? Why have I been the recipient of many good things and she has much trouble? This plagues me at times when I observe the hardship of her young twenty-four-year-old life. The only answer must be is that I have experienced undeserved *grace*.

Today, my niece and her husband received their new daughter from India. She is two years old and weighs fourteen pounds. Clothing for a one-year-old is too big for her. This little girl is one of many, many orphans from a vastly populated country. She was literally delivered to a home that will be like a palace to her. Why was she picked versus another child in the orphanage? What could an abandoned infant do to deserve the extravagant care she will now receive in a foreign country by strangers who paid for her, sight unseen?

Her new parents will lavish her with love. From a woven mat on a floor to a pink bedroom with a soft mattress and clean sheets, she will sleep in the comfort of a princess. She has experienced the miracle of being chosen by *grace*.

My friend Sasha was once an orphan too. Also from India, her parents adopted her twenty four years ago. Her American father regularly performed therapy on her legs which were afflicted with rickets, a result of malnourishment in the orphanage. He was a chiropractor. She was blessed to be an adopted child of a physician who could meet her individual need for this type of care. She experienced being chosen by *grace*.

We, too, have been chosen and adopted into God's family through no merit of our own. "It is by grace you have been saved and not that of yourselves, it is a gift from God—not by works so no one can boast" *Ephesians 2:9*.

And why would he do this for such as us? We were sinners, dead in our transgressions like the rest. "It is by grace you have been saved. And God raised us up with Christ and seated us with him in the heavenly realms in Christ Jesus, in order that in the coming ages he might show the incomparable riches of his grace, expressed in his kindness to us in Jesus Christ" *Ephesians 2: 6*.

We were as poor orphans, destitute and abandoned. He walked into our lives and took us up in his arms and brought us to his table and his home. Now he cares for us, provides for us, and loves us.

Today I wondered how my niece's new daughter reacted to her father. You see, my niece's husband is a very tall man, with dark hair, dark eyes, and could possibly appear like a giant to a small child. From the reports we've received, she went to him gladly. We call him the "gentle giant." His gentleness is one attribute that towers over his physical height.

This to me is a beautiful picture of Christ's love for us. He is huge, powerful, Lord of all creation and heaven. He is a king. Mortals and demons tremble at his name and his presence. Yet he is a humble king; he stoops to conquer. He said, "Come unto me, all you who are weary and burdened, and I will give you rest. Take my yoke upon you and learn from me, for I am *gentle and humble* in heart…and you will find rest for your souls" Matt.

11:28. We, like children, can give ourselves to him and not fear.

Chosen by grace. He chose us, we didn't choose him. We will sit at the king's table and enjoy an inheritance that we didn't deserve or have any right to. We are the adopted children of the most beloved King that has ever been or will ever be.

Let that thought infuse your mind. Muse on the joy that is to come when we enter eternity. Saturate your soul with thoughts of gratitude to the One who chose you. The lyrics to this song by Harriet E. Buell, (1877), say it all.

A CHILD OF THE KING

Yes, Oh Yes,
I'm a Child of the King,
His royal blood now flows through my veins,
And I who was wretched and poor, now can sing,
Praise God, Praise God,
I'm a child of the King….

My Father is rich in houses and lands.
He holdeth the wealth of the world in his hands!
Of rubies and diamonds, of silver and gold,
His coffers are full, He has riches untold.

GRACE INFUSIONS

My Father's own Son, the Savior of men,
Once wandered on earth as the poorest of them;
But now He is pleading our pardon on high,
That we may be His, when He comes by and by.

I once was an outcast stranger on earth,
A sinner by choice, an alien by birth,
But I've been adopted, my name's written down,
An heir to a mansion, a robe and a crown.

A tent or a cottage, why should I care?
They're building a palace for me over there;
Though exiled from home, yet still may I sing;
All glory to God, I'm a child of the king.

Grace on the Job

New Nurses Need Grace

Making a medication error was the worst thing a nurse could ever do. At least this is what I thought after having J. Stephenson as a pharmacology instructor. And then it happened.

A few months after I was hired for my first job as a nurse, I did it. I made my first error in a pediatric clinic where eight physicians saw approximately one hundred kids a day. I'll never forget it.

It was about 4:30 p.m., nearing the end of our day. Three phones rang incessantly at our work station especially at that time of day, with mothers wanting antibiotics for kids with earaches, or nurses at the hospital trying to contact one of our many doctors for orders.

I had been running the halls checking in patients, weighing babies, giving immunizations and all the other things pediatric nurses do. Suddenly I stopped dead in my tracks at the med counter. I realized I had just made a serious mistake. My heart pounded at the idea--I couldn't think clearly.

When it occurred to me that I may have made an error I went to my boss immediately and informed her of my questionable mistake. I had possibly injected wrong medication into the arm of an asthmatic infant. I became even more upset when my young supervisor threw up her hands, backed away and said, "You're on your own! Go tell Eichner."

On my own? I'm a new nurse! You are my supervisor with experience, not to mention my best friend at work.... *on my own?* Anxiety rose up in me like the Incredible Hulk bursting out of his mortal clothes. It threatened to overtake me. Being abandoned in a time of crisis is not what I had expected and yet here I was: alone to deal with my mistake, worried about my little patient, and my job security---alone to deal with the humiliation of doing the most awful thing a nurse could do (At least in my mind.)

I went to Dr. Eichner who ordered the injection, and told him I thought I possibly gave the wrong medication to this child. He said, "Let's think about this for a moment." He was calm, logical, and his usual easygoing self. We deduced that, in fact, I had given the wrong medication and he instructed me to go give the right drug and explain to the parents what had happened.

With dignity and respect I told the parents what I had done, apologized, and asked them if they minded me giving the correct medication to their daughter. Thankfully, they were gracious to me, and I administered the right med to the little girl.

Directly after doing the right thing in this wrong situation, I went to the break room, flopped on a bean bag chair and started sobbing. My emotional kettle was boiling over from the stress of my error and the fear of causing harm to a child. The tears poured from my eyes, my chest was aching and heaving with relief and distress at the same time if that's even possible. Suddenly the door to the room opened and there stood Dr. Eichner.

"Are you okay?" he said with a gentle smile.

I buried my head in the bag and waved him away as I was uncontrollably crying.

That evening after musing about the day's events and talking with my husband who is also a nurse, I came to the conclusion that all nurses make mistakes. We are only human and mistakes will happen. I was not the worst nurse in the world. And chances are that one day in the future it would happen again and, therefore, I decided to make peace with myself.

The next morning Dr. Eichner entered the office as usual with his briefcase in one hand and a coffee cup in the other. Our eyes met and he said, "Are you done brow beating yourself yet?" His kindness infused me.

I said, "Yep." And it was over. No more hashing it out, no more brutalizing myself, no more harsh thoughts about being the worst nurse on the planet, no more anger at myself. I gave myself grace. Dr. Eichner offered me grace. It was over. Yesterday was gone.

My boss, well, I had to offer her grace for not being able to be there for me in a time of need. She is human, too, and a nurse. And she made a mistake.

Grace on the job. We all need it now and then. Take it when you need it. Give it when someone else needs it. Especially to those young novices who are learning. And to those who are stressed (are there any who aren't?!)

Timely Grace

God's grace is always right on time

Hugging the side of the road, I approached a hill and veered around a sharp curve. Suddenly an SUV came rushing toward me over the center line. I jerked my truck to the right to get out of its direct trajectory, not looking to see if there was a tree or anything in the path. I just wanted to get out its path immediately.

Thankfully, that last minute horn blast and dart off the road saved me from a head on collision; or was it timely grace? I'd say I was saved by grace at that moment because I could have slammed into a tree or pole in the densely wooded area to my right.

Twenty six years prior to this incident, I was thrown off the back of a motorcycle at just about midnight on this same road, very close to where this near-accident occurred. In a terrifying instant, I was tumbling through the darkness. It was literally so black around me that I could not see my hand in front of my face. Disoriented, I began screaming hysterically.

Also dazed by what had just happened, my husband appeared out of nowhere and grabbed me. He, too, was tossed off the bike when we missed a curve in the darkness and he went head over heels with the bike down the road.

Being in the total darkness is very scary even when you have your wits about you. It's more frightening when you are compromised physically, mentally, or emotionally. It elicits panic from way down deep inside.

After assessing our injuries, we were taken to the hospital for treatment. My husband was admitted for a severed patellar tendon on his leg just below the knee. I had gravel scrubbed out of the heel of a foot and elbow and was sent home to our three-year-old son on crutches. I had to get back to nursing school that week or I'd be out of the program. No absenteeism was allowed for any reason so I hobbled the next few weeks to and from class, books and all.

TIMELY GRACE

Three days after my husband had surgery on his leg, I received an urgent phone call to come to the hospital. The nursing supervisor of the hospital took me into an office and told me that my husband was transferred to ICU for a pulmonary embolism and that he may not survive the event. I sat there in disbelief as they talked to me about being prepared for the worst.

I couldn't even go see him after they informed me of the gravity of his situation; I wasn't allowed in the ICU. They sent me home. I gimped on my crutches and went back home. I cried. I lay awake in the bed all night racked with anxiety. *I was too young to be a widow. What if he died? What about our little boy?*

We hadn't exactly been living right. The night of the motorcycle accident my husband had had a few drinks with friends when he picked me up. I couldn't pray with any confidence of God's hearing or help because I knew how our lives really were. We argued too much, partied too much, and, though we did have a measure of faith in God, we were very immature in so many ways.

I knew this situation was out of my control. I felt more in the dark now than the night I was in the woods screaming. Life and death are in God's control. I didn't even feel I had the right to pray and ask God to keep my husband alive.

During my husband's days in the ICU, he was afraid to go to sleep lest he not wake up. He felt the presence of death around him and was in pain, but didn't want the nurse to medicate him for fear he wouldn't wake up. He felt guilty about his own behaviors and didn't feel close to God. He was deeply distressed inwardly, and very anxious about living or dying.

While lying in his hospital bed one afternoon, a volunteer delivered mail to him. On the front of the card was the large hand of a man, with a newborn infant in its palm. It read, "Don't worry, God is holding you in the palm of his hand. With love from your friends at your grandmother's church. Ever since we heard of your accident, we have not stopped praying for you." He wept. The fear of death vanished and the peace of God flooded his heart and he knew that he was not beyond the strong reach of God's hand. A timely reminder of grace in his hour of need was delivered at just the right moment.

What a picture of God's grace. He holds us in his hand. He holds us when we're bad, and when we're good. He holds us in his hand when we're young and immature, and when we're old and gray. He holds us.

Isaiah describes this very promise of being held by our heavenly Father. "But Zion said, "The Lord has forsaken me, the Lord has forgotten me. Can a mother forget the baby at her breast and have no compassion on the child she has bore? Though she may forget, I will not forget you. See, I have engraved you on the palms of my hands" Isa 49:16 NIV.

Recently I was diagnosed with carpal tunnel syndrome in my right hand. I notice that my grip is not what it used to be. Yesterday I dropped the dog food container and kibbles scattered all over my kitchen floor. Later that night, I flung a knife across the room because my grip is no longer functioning properly! Human hands and human strength fail! God's grip on his children never fails. He *never* lets go. Through the calm and through the storms of life, he never ever lets go. And his grace is always right on time…..

Grace for Patients and Patience

Give it. Take it. Share it. Grace.

I called the patient's name for his scheduled appointment and a double wide wheelchair with a very large man in it rolled toward me. I had never seen a double wide wheelchair before and was caught off guard by my own thoughts.

I was already exasperated by my difficult coworkers at my new position in this clinic and it was only 9 o'clock in the morning. I wasn't in the mood to deal with a difficult patient *or* a patient with difficulties.

I'd already called the man's name and as he entered the hallway I knew he would not fit into my small exam room where I did work-ups before patients saw the eye doctor. Anxiously I sought out another that had a chair large enough to accommodate him and hoped it would work for both of us.

Earlier that morning I'd been provoked by two co-workers who took some of my required equipment out of my exam room. I'd already had to confront one of them just before I started the exam on this particular patient. I didn't know why this pair seemed to enjoy tormenting me. Possibly it was because I was a Christian, but, whatever the reason, it was painful to me and more irritating than sandpaper on fair skin.

My face probably shouted "distress" in body language as I began my usual ophthalmic work up on this man.

The gentle giant reached out his hand to me before we began and asked, "May I pray for you?"

I was shocked and humbled. Only seconds before his offer, I had thoughts of racing out of the building and never returning. I felt more out of place than with any other job I've ever had.

I held his hand, and with the exam room door wide open in a non-Christian environment, we bowed our heads. He prayed one of the most meaningful prayers for me that anyone had ever prayed. I was stunned at his sensitivity to my anguish, though he had no idea of what had been going on in that office. The strife and conflict had worn me down. I felt all alone in a place where I didn't feel wanted or accepted. I was receiving a *grace infusion* through his prayer and reassuring touch.

He looked at me with deep compassion. He knew nothing about me but was reading my emotional mail and ministering to my hurting heart.

He offered grace. I thanked him then and sent him a thank you note many days later.

I felt very sorrowful for my initial uneasy thoughts about his size, and was deeply repentant when he offered me life-saving grace and kindness in my moment of need. I was reminded that I need to give my patients grace. Grace when they are unkind. Grace when they are different than my expectations. Grace when they are suffering in their own unique way. Grace, grace, grace. I need to give it lavishly as Jesus has so lavished his love upon us.

Thinking of this incident is a reminder of another. This was again in an office where I prepared patients to see an eye doctor, but it was in a different office environment entirely. I was surrounded by Christian co-workers in this work place. It was one of the best places I ever worked and I have fond memories of being there.

I scanned the waiting room as I reviewed my next patient's chart. I was really hoping that it was not the guy in leathers, tattoos, and dark glasses. I am a conservative, somewhat timid kind of a girl. As I looked at his age I knew that *he* was my man. Everyone else in the room was over 65 and he was under 30.

I called out the name and the biker sauntered toward me. We entered the exam room and the first thing he says is, "You probably think I'm a drug addict. I'm not. I'm a born again Christian."

Quite honestly, he was right. I had already reviewed his chart and noted that he had a liver transplant and was on a ton of medications that organ transplant patients typically take. I did think he probably had pickled his liver with alcohol or dirty needles.

"I got a miracle," he proceeded to tell me. "I was the last person on the list to receive a liver, and I got a miracle."

He told me his story. At one point, he was eating Tylenol like candy for serious back pain. He ended up in the E.R. with flu-like symptoms and was diagnosed with liver failure from chronic over usage of Tylenol. We've all the heard the warnings. It's a fact; too much acetaminophen will destroy your liver.

I have back pain; I understand. I just recently had two sets of steroid injections in my lower back for pain. I also take pain medication routinely for it. I understand his pain.

He then told me that he and his Christian biker friends ride for "Bibles in China." They get thousands of donated Bibles to send overseas to China. He was truly an inspiration and I loved talking with him. Again, I needed to be reminded that no matter what my patients look like, they need grace.

One of my co-workers asked him what he thought about Jesus' command to "turn the other cheek" and what he would do if someone "jumped him."

"I'd kick their ass," he replied.

Laughing out loud, we gave him grace! Even bikers need grace and sanctification-- and we know that's God's work—not ours! Grace for patients— God's good grace. Share it. Show it. Give it. Spread it. Love it. Amazing grace!

Grace for the Dying

Do not let your hearts be troubled.....

John 14:27

Being a hospice nurse late in my nursing career allowed me to be at the bedside of many in their final days, hours and moments. I was blessed to share grace with both strangers *and* people that I knew well.

As a very young nurse, entering the room of a dead patient or being with a patient who was terminally ill was a frightening thought to me. I was not comfortable with death. We didn't talk about it in our home as I grew up. It was one of those *unspoken rules*. My father died when I was twenty years old. He had cancer of the liver and stomach and his health declined rapidly over approximately eight months. He breathed his last in the icy month of February, 1978.

GRACE INFUSIONS

I was only weeks away from birthing our son, Benjamin, when he was diagnosed. Months before my father had seen the surgeon, he appeared weak and not his usual self. I sensed there was something terribly wrong and my husband and I prayed for him in our alone times, and I wept a lot. I sensed impending doom.

One of my sweetest memories with him was at our summer cottage on Clear Lake the summer before he passed. I would lie on the fold out couch with my arm around him. No words were needed. I was great with child and he referred to me as the "Michelin Man" more than once during my pregnancy, though I had no idea what he meant! I saw the commercial months after he was gone and laughed at his picture of me as a giant with tires around my middle! I did look that way, as most full term pregnancies do!

One of my saddest memories is when the morticians arrived at my parents' home, and my younger brothers and I were asked to go into one of the bedrooms and shut the door while they removed his remains from the home he'd built for us eleven years before. A horrible silence filled the house. I ached to comfort my brothers and to be comforted but, as I recall, we didn't speak a word.

GRACE FOR THE DYING

We didn't talk about his illness or his death as a family. Silence was our maladaptive coping skill as passed down through generations. We were stoic. We didn't complain when we were ill or in pain. We didn't talk about our feelings. By example, we learned to *"put up and shut up."* To be weak was to be less and was looked upon unfavorably.

It is no wonder that, as a young nurse, I abhorred the idea of being with the dying patient. But as time went by, I grew and matured. My faith in God grew, especially in my thirties. I was baptized at age 32 and made a public declaration to be a disciple of Jesus. It felt wonderful and I desired to learn more about the Bible and prayer.

At about age 41, I started caring for patients with Alzheimer's disease. I watched the progression of the disease over months or even years while they were under my care. I attended at the bedside and watched the mystery of the end of life unfold again and again in this memory care facility. It is here where I transitioned to hospice nursing.

One of my most memorable patients was a forty-year-old woman with breast cancer. She also had one of the most obvious and debilitating cases of depression I'd ever seen. Her facial countenance was as flat as the tiled floor in her ward room. She spoke haltingly. She moved slowly. Depression had afflicted her for many years even before the cancer invaded her life.

I had the pleasure of taking her out of the facility one afternoon to see her husband, and then the two of us stopped at a local café for a piece of pie. After we enjoyed our pie, she gingerly took long drags on a cigarette and sipped on her coffee. It was one of her last outings. We celebrated together the simple joys of life. On the way back to the nursing home we sat by the river and talked about her life. She loved to sew and tenderly reminisced about her mother. We then held hands together and prayed aloud---each of us. Grace filled the air as we beseeched God to be near.

Her parents were both deceased and her husband was in a group home as he was paraplegic and also had mental afflictions, leaving him unable to care for himself. She was now living out her time in a nursing home. It tore at my heart for her to be dying, so alone in the world. One of our goals as a hospice team was to be nearby when the time came. And her time came when I happened to be on duty.

My young patient was barely conscious and not moving; her breathing slowed and became more shallow by the second. I knew the dying process can take hours and I felt pressured to visit my other patients in the facility that day. I gave up that thought and pulled up a geri-chair and settled in for the long haul. After I reclined, I grabbed my patient's hand and resolved that she would *not be alone at the very end.*

A sweet nurse's aide entered the room some time later and we both held hands over her and prayed as she breathed her last breath. It was over.

I went to make my necessary phone calls to her husband and the mortuary. Upon returning to her room, the woman appeared most beautiful, as if in restful slumber. This young woman appeared cherub-like. Her face was still puffy from steroids but something was different. There was a childlikeness in her countenance and a peace that washed away her depressive affect. It was quite remarkable and touching. The next day our team chaplain made the same observation when he went to her memorial service. "She looked like a cherub," he said.

Jesus comforts us with his words to his disciples. "Do not let your hearts be troubled. Trust in God; trust also in me. In my Father's house are many rooms; if it were not so, I would have told you. I am going there to prepare a place for you, I will come back and take you to be with me that you also may be where I am" John 14:1-4 NIV.

"Peace I leave with you; my peace I give you. I do not give to you as the world gives. Do not let your hearts be afraid" John 14:27 NIV.

Grace for the dying. Be available. Be gracious. Just be there. This is grace in action. Pray for the dying, pray with the dying. Pray for grace. Infuse someone with loving care.

Grace for the Race

I am not a runner. I hate running. I love swimming but hate running. It takes away my breath and jars my feet, knees and hips. It hurts my back too.

I envy my 40-something-year-old sister in law. She is a runner. She wasn't always a runner but she is now and I'm proud of her! She participates in marathons and finishes the races she starts.

We are all going to finish this race of life one way or the other and some of us sooner than others. I knew a woman who was 60 when she started running. She actually participated in a 26-mile run and I am still amazed at her!

Well, the life race has been compared to a marathon in more than one book. And I think of this as I watch my mother, who is 86, struggling in this life race. She walks with a walker now and at times easily tires at the store when shopping. I think of this as my frail aunt 'runs' her race with Alzheimer's

GRACE INFUSIONS

Disease and failing health at the age of 89. She can no longer walk but is now in a wheelchair.

When my mom received word that a friend of ours had passed after many years of Alzheimer's soon after she made a visit to my aunt in a memory care facility, she almost quit life's race herself. She dropped out of the race and into her recliner chair for a whole day. Shedding tears on and off, she was unable to shake the sadness that exhausted her heart.

How can I revive her heart? How can I encourage her? I was troubled and felt helpless as I saw her vitality vanish and knew the pain with which she was struggling.

The next day I pulled out an old tape player and picked out some good cassettes from a church she liked. As I mowed the lawn and she endeavored to do the dishes, I played the tape for her.

Later on, she sat on the porch swing while I finished doing some much needed yard work and I put I my IPOD ear phones in her good ear to let her listen to some more worship music. I gave her spirit an infusion! Her countenance was brightened and she appeared at peace instead of distressed and heavyhearted. I even heard her humming to the music.

GRACE FOR THE RACE

She gave me a hug and a kiss. "I love you, Mary," she said. "This is what I need. " And she held me close.

Physical touch, hearing the Word of God, and worship music: a good remedy for tired runners in this race of life. Hook someone up to a grace infusion. There is someone near you in need of one....

Isaiah 40:29-31 NIV

He gives strength to the weary and increases the power of the weak. Even youths grow tired and weary, and young men stumble and fall; but those who hope in the Lord will renew their strength. They will soar on wings like eagles; they will run and not grow weary, they will walk and not faint.

Amen?

Indescribable Grace

I'd been putting it off for months. Don't ask me why. I knew I should stop by the Christian bookstore and return the DVDs I'd checked out from the video library. Days went by. Then months. Then even more than a year! As time increased with the overdue DVDs, so did my anxiety and embarrassment over having had them *way too long*!

Now I *had* to return them because I was to do a book signing at this very store in one month and I was mortified! Time was squeezing me tighter each day so I gathered my courage and prepared myself to eat a huge piece of humble pie. I prayed for grace while dashing across the street to the store to face the music.

"I am so mortified! I'm so embarrassed. I can hardly look at you!" I rambled on to the sweet store owner.

Pointing her finger, smiling, and trying to

search for words, she spouted, "Oh, it was you!" And then she laughed. "I was trying to remember who had those and where we got the idea to look at them."

Oh thank God she couldn't remember that it was procrastinator me! Her smile melted away the fear that had kept me frozen and away from her store for months.

"I'm so sorry!" I went on.

Then she said something I never expected: "Because you told me about the "Indescribable" DVD by Louie Gigglio, my husband showed it to his men's Bible study group. We sold 30 copies of it. We never would have if you didn't tell us about it!

I felt infused with an indescribable grace at that moment. God made something very good out of some not-so-good behavior and despite my propensity to procrastinate! Instead of being disgusted with me, she appeared thrilled.

Next, this sincere lady confessed one of her own blunders to comfort me. I sensed her sincere care and open heart to God and to me. I was truly blessed. The guilt lifted off my shoulders and my heart, peace settled back on them, and my spirit was strengthened by her grace infusion. I paid for the DVD's and my debt was cancelled.

If you want to be infused to your very core, get the DVD "Indescribable." Have some friends over and view it together. Prepare to be infused beyond your wildest imagination as Louie Gigglio takes you on a tour through our galaxy and actual photos from the Hubble telescope. Psalm 19 says it perfectly, "The universe displays the glory of God and there is no place on earth where their voice is not heard!" NIV

"Indescribable, uncontainable, you placed the stars in the sky and you call them by name! You are amazing, God!

A Place in Need of Grace

A Hospital Not So Far Away

Can you imagine a hospital with no sheets on a
bed; no pillow to lay your head?
No call light to call for help.
A hospital with blood on the floor; rooms without a door,
Where someone lies shivering, shaking, face down
on concrete- a place where nothing looks neat.
A hospital with no air conditioning when it's 100
degrees; where babies with pneumonia can hardly
breathe;
A pharmacy with no pills, bottles, or IVs; this
place diagnosed with hopelessness as an incurable
disease.
A hospital with newborn babies with no baby fat,
thrust into poverty; just think of that.
No carts, dinner trays, or cafeterias here; but a

man selling oranges on the street.
It doesn't appear there is much here to eat.
This hospital I have seen, not in my imagination,
but in a city of 150,000 in a very poor nation.
Are we really our brothers' keeper? Has the message Jesus gave to "go into *all* the world" become
cheaper?
Lord, please help us to love-not with words or
with tongue; but with actions and truth. Lead us
now to pick up our cross and follow you.

I wrote this poem only hours after visiting this hospital on a medical mission trip. I was stunned, shocked, and dismayed after the tour. There was no grace to be found in this place. At least I didn't see it, so I figured it didn't exist.

Tears poured down my cheeks as I observed women in labor on beds with no sheets, pads or towels. A surgical patient was wrapped in a blanket that looked as though it had been retrieved from a landfill. Water dripped from above through stained and missing ceiling tiles right over the pre-op scrub sink. There was absolutely no grace in this place.

I take it back. There was some grace. It was embodied in our tour guide who was a lab technician at the hospital. He proudly showed us each ward and even the Emergency Room. His smile was calming. His stride was confident. This was where he worked every day and he graced this far away place. He was kind and gentle; a caring person. Just the kind of person you'd want to take care of you at any hospital.

The nurses in their secondhand uniforms greeted us warmly. No hosiery needed in this tropical environment, and most wore sandals. Their hair, pulled back in simple pony tails was the only evident appearance of "professionalism." It was oddly silent throughout this hospital. No overhead speakers blaring Code Blue announcements or asking doctors to pick up line one. No IV pumps beeping incessantly or phones ringing non-stop. No bed alarms clanging; just dead silence.

A dog roamed the halls like he owned the place, scavenging for anything. There was nothing to be found, however. No one seemed disturbed by the stray animals roving in and out of the hospital freely. To see a mangy canine running free in this place to treat the ill distressed me. Who knows what disease it carried in with it?

I was relieved to get back on our bus and head to our very modest but clean hotel. I couldn't shake the visions of sick people on the army green vinyl mattresses and a handwritten sign on the wall that said, "CHOLERA." These particular patients had beds with holes in the mattress, strategically placed, and pans on the floor under them for their special needs.

I collapsed on my bed and tried to shut out the visions of the afternoon tour, but it was overwhelming. My mind and heart had been traumatized. The extreme poverty was revolting to me. I couldn't accept that this was their best care in a huge city but it was reality.

I felt like I needed an infusion---of what I wasn't sure. My cold shower with a gecko looking on didn't help much. Singing and fellowshipping later that evening with my missionary friends didn't do it. As I reflect on this, I went back to America feeling despondent over what I had witnessed in this poor nation. I had been changed by what I perceived as a shortage of grace in this far away place.

I've seen movies where some people returning to the U.S.A. have bowed and kissed the soil. Those thoughts infiltrated my mind as our plane landed back in Houston. "God bless America, land that I love…." flowed through my heart and mind on the flight home. I had a true sense of gratitude for my country and the grace that God has shed on it. I experienced a humbling sense of gratitude because I was born here. I didn't merit the blessing; I could have been born where I just witnessed thousands of people residing--- 80% in dire poverty.

Grace in a faraway place. Sometimes one has to look carefully for it and sometimes we are the ones who should grace the places we visit. Be open to being a grace giver—a grace goer—and a grace infuser in a foreign setting.

Carrying Grace

In all their distress he, too, was distressed and the angel of his presence saved them. In his love and mercy he redeemed them. He lifted them up and carried them.

Isaiah 63:9

When was the last time someone carried you? I mean literally, carried you? Take a moment and think about this.

The last time I remember someone carrying me was my father when I was in the third grade. He carried me out of our house, into the car, and then into the hospital where he finally laid me in a bed on the Pediatric Ward. I was nine years old.

Earlier that particular day I fell ill at school. I could not keep my head off my desk and just lay in a heap over it. My sweet teacher took my hand and led me to the office and called my mother at work to come get me.

My mom whisked me off to the doctor's office where I received a shot of penicillin in my behind and then went next door to the hospital for labs and chest x-ray. I remember being too tired and weak to even talk.

Later after a few hours at home, I heard the phone ring. The doctor informed my mother that I needed to be admitted and to bring me to the hospital.

My father, a carpenter by trade, still in his cement-splashed khakis, white tee shirt and work boots came quietly down the hallway to my room and picked me up in his arms. This alarmed me though I didn't show it. I was nine years old, not two. I was nervous about the car ride and the idea of going to a hospital. But I felt totally safe in his arms. I was completely weak and he was completely strong. His biceps bulged even when he was at rest. His hands were strong and big, with tough calluses on them.

As I reflect on this memory, I cannot help but think of my heavenly Father. I think of Jesus, who said, "If you've seen me, you've seen the Father." Jesus was a carpenter, too, and no doubt was physically strong. Many who were sick were brought to him for healing. He also went to those who were sick and dying before he was ever asked to. Isaiah 53:4 states, "Surely he took up our infirmities and *carried* our sorrows."

Infirmities are physical weaknesses or ailments, especially because of age or an unsteady mind. It can mean a moral failure or weakness as well.

When we battle illnesses or mental and emotional difficulties, it is comforting to know that Jesus himself took up our infirmities and carried our sorrows, because it is a reality for each of us sometime in our lives.

During times of weakness, we still need to trust in Jesus as a child, with childlike faith. Jesus said, "Let the little children come to me and do not hinder them, for the kingdom of heaven belongs to such as these" Matt. 19:14.

That day my father walked into my room and lifted me in his arms, I didn't call for him. I didn't even know he was coming. He knew, though, that I was weak and could not help myself. I didn't have to call for him; he came to me.

I will muse over the picture of my loving, strong father carrying me and will cherish the memory all of my life. I will think of how my heavenly Father came to earth in the form of a man, Jesus, and how he carried a heavy cross upon which he was crucified so that I may be healed and my sins forgiven. He came to earth for each of us; when we were too sick to call out for him, he came to us. He continues to carry us when we are alone and hurting, or sick and dying. He is full of "carrying" grace.

> *I have upheld you since you were conceived and have carried you since birth. Even to your old age and gray hairs, I am he. I am he who will sustain you. I have made you and I will carry you. I will sustain you and I will rescue you.*
>
> *Isaiah 46: 3-*

Grace at Your Own Pace

Strip down, start running—and never quit! No extra spiritual fat, no parasitic sins. Keep your eyes on Jesus, who both began and finished this race we're in. Study how he did it. Because he never lost sight of where he was headed—that exhilarating finish in and with God—he could put up with anything along the way; cross, shame, whatever. And now he's there, in the place of honor, right alongside the Father. When you find yourself flagging in your faith, go over that story again, item by item, that long litany of hostility he plowed through. That will shoot adrenaline into your soul!

Heb 12:1 The Message / / Remix / Peterson

Focused on the black line, stretching each stroke, and breathing on the count of three is my goal in the pool three times a week for thirty minutes. Face down, then face to the side, breathe and back down, I concentrate on my rhythm and look ahead for the cross emblem stationed at each end of the lane under the surface of the water. I know I'm almost there when I glimpse the cross.

Then it happens. The Olympic swimmer-type gets in the lane next to me and speeds past me and suddenly my rhythm is interrupted. My focused, fifty-year-old swimmer self is instantly out of breath and I no longer have the black line in sight beneath me but am disoriented, gasping like a fish out of water. My steady pace is totally disturbed now, and it feels like I was accosted by the pace of another.

I peer through my steamed goggles to see if I can spot the end of the lane. I glance over the roped lane to see if the sleek shark is already turning around and heading back toward me. I tell myself *it doesn't matter* that I swim slower, and yet I am oddly distracted and feel less fit, almost discouraged.

Before the Olympian entered the water, I felt like an Olympian myself. Then I see the younger, fit, and powerful swimmer and I almost drown in feelings of inadequacy and 'water worthlessness' in my attempts to swim at my own pace.

Why do we humans do this? Compare one

another? Compare ourselves to others? It's a meaningless and harmful game we play when we entertain thoughts of trying to "measure up." Whether in the pool, in school, in the church, or on the job, we are apt to fall into this meaningless trap.

Before I begin to sink into depths of self pity or self depreciating thoughts at the pool, I shake off the anxious thoughts and try to recompose my focus once again on my goal. Exercising my body, for my health, for my well being, for thirty minutes, three times a week: that's it. Accepting myself as a fifty-year-old, looking more middle-aged than ever, some pounds overweight, I cut myself some slack---grace to grow older at my own pace and grace to swim laps at my own pace; not another's.

I used to think I should be more spiritual, and I should have achieved more life goals by this age, and I look at others around me and fall into that snare of comparison. I still have goals and dreams unfulfilled and probably will no matter how long I live. We all will. What matters is that we go and grow at our own pace. God is watching. He knows our frames our desires and our dreams. He promises to finish what he has started in us; he knows the right pace. He has set the pace for us as individuals.

GRACE INFUSIONS

Persevering and *keeping on keeping on* is the goal. It's not how fast or slow we go; it's going on in spite of difficulties, distractions, trials, temptations and in spite of how fast or slow our neighbor is moving. We need to fix our eyes on Jesus; he is our goal, keeping our eyes on the cross, despising the suffering, and accepting the sovereignty of God. He will give us grace to go at our correct pace.

Forgiving Grace

Forgive us our trespasses as we forgive those who trespass against us.

Mat. 6:14

I couldn't believe it. They wouldn't pray for me. My dearest friends in ministry turning their backs on me because I was invited to go on a medical mission trip overseas. Jesus said to "go into all the world," and I wanted to obey. But why should believers in Christ not want me to obey him at his call?

This disturbed me and caused me some of the most severe innermost anguish I've ever experienced. I was shunned, to put it politely, when I told my ministry leader that I was invited by my physician friend to fill a much needed spot on a trip to Borneo. That spot was already paid for, and, at the last moment, the person who was supposed to go was unable to.

Oddly, almost unbelievably, I'd had a dream weeks prior to this phone call. I was on a huge plane with two men with whom I worked previously at an eye clinic in the States. We had tons of stuff with us too. I remember vividly thinking in the dream: *Are we going to India?* Now living in Arizona, it was even stranger to get a call from former co-workers in Michigan, specifically requesting me to go to Borneo with them to do cataract surgery in a poor jungle village hospital for two weeks.

Being the mission-minded person I am, I didn't need a lot of time to decide whether to go or not. My boss at the time was a Christian, and our executive director was in Haiti on a mission trip to build a school or church when I asked for the two weeks off to go. The door was wide open.

I made the decision to go with my husband's blessing as well. Flying for 24 hours to get to a place 10,000 miles from home was not particularly romantic, especially our last flight from Singapore to Pontianak, on the island of Borneo. We couldn't land because of smoke from seasonal burning of rice fields. So we circled the airstrip for forty five long, hot, sickening minutes. The aircraft was like a roller coaster; the heat from the equator caused us to make dips and rises as we went around and around the airport below.

The girl next to me grabbed her little bag from the back of the seat in front of her; I felt nauseous and grabbed mine too. Row by row, the heaving started from the front of the jet all the way to the back. Air sickness infiltrated the sixty-passenger plane all at once. We landed moments after the tossing of many cookies!

The passengers handed off their gross packages to the flight attendants as we deplaned. The heat from the equator hit me in the face like a furnace blowing at me in fifty-mile-an-hour gusts. I was too hot to be nauseated anymore and we hopped into a small car with no seatbelts for a five-hour ride into the jungle.

Not being in the car more than fifteen minutes; I let out a scream as I saw a guy on the motor bike heading right at my side of the vehicle. My physician friend said, "MB, just cover your face!" The traffic was nightmarish and chaotic. I did just what he said and took a small pillow and hid my eyes behind it. Thankfully, I was so tired from the air travel that I fell asleep in the car most of the way to our final destination.

GRACE INFUSIONS

This particular medical mission turned out to be one of the hardest but best mission trips I'd ever been on. We worked long hours at a little village hospital where all the women were under five feet tall and weighed about eighty pounds. The men weren't much taller and were very slight in build. Everywhere we looked we saw dark tanned skin and dark brown irises. They were from the Dayak tribe in this part of West Kalimantan.

Each day after our work was done and after meal time I would retire to my small room which consisted of a single mattress on a slab frame about four feet off the floor, a wardrobe closet, a table and chair, a sink, and small bathroom.

The bathing accommodations were just as I'd heard. A tiled and cement tank holding many gallons of river water was about four feet high by three feet wide. A red plastic bowl with a handle on it sat on the rim, and a drain in the floor was nearby.

To bathe, one must use the red bowl and dip into the fresh water tank and pour it over one's head several times to get wet; then soap up and rinse with more water. It is quite shocking to the system when one's body temperature outside is the same as the equatorial degrees! The water was not heated but after about two to three bowls of water the shock turns to a pleasing cool rinse, a relief from the intense jungle heat.

I reflected on the day's work and wrote in my journal. Thoughts of America would slip into my mind and again I would feel the angst of being rejected by my dear friends back home. The anger would rise; the disillusionment of being in ministry, and a sort of despair would creep in because I knew I wouldn't be in the jungle forever and I'd have to face them again soon.

I read my Bible, looking for some comfort and some way to deal with the intense inner feelings regarding the ordeal before my departure. I was racked with anxiety, wondering how to handle this awful, public situation.

A little wooden, hand-painted sign was the only wall hanging in my room. I would stare at it and try to figure out its meaning. It appeared to be a scripture verse that looked like this: Rum 12,

One morning, I yanked the sign off the wall above my bed and brought it with me to breakfast where four of us ate together daily. An American fellow ate with us every day though he was on an independent mission, having grown up in the area. I knew he could tell me the mystery of this unfamiliar language that seemed to nag at me every day in my room.

I held up the sign. "What does this say?"

"Do good to those who do evil to you," he politely replied. It was from the book of Romans, chapter 12, verse 21 that states, "Do not be overcome by evil, but overcome evil with good."

My countenance fell, if not outwardly, then inwardly.

Do good to the people back home who refused to even pray for me or wish me well as I trekked ten thousand miles from home? Do good to them who turned their backs on me? Do good to those who accosted my heart with so much emotional distress and pain? My mind ranted over this concept and I didn't like it. I had been praying for wisdom and guidance about the situation; this was not the answer I'd expected. I knew it was God speaking to me though, and I started to muse on that.

Jesus opened not his mouth against those who taunted him, saying, "So you are the King of the Jews, are you?" In the next breath they called him Beelzebub and worse.

I wanted to run my mouth against my friends. I wanted to vindicate myself and defend myself; but that was not what God was instructing me to do. He wanted me to not open my mouth against these dear friends who had taunted me. I asked him for grace and more grace because I knew I couldn't do it on my own.

While shopping in a nearby city for things to bring home to loved ones from this very extraordinary island country, I deliberately picked some items to bring back to my ministry friends. Baked goods such as cookies, Indonesian candy, and beautiful beaded pen jackets were some of the things I found. I was taking God at his word and trying to "do good."

Our mission trip ended with our goals being met: new friends and relationships made, and a unique jungle part of God's world became planted in my heart.

After twenty eight hours and eight separate flights to get back to the U.S., I arrived home to my husband who watched me sleep for fifteen hours non-stop. Jet lag and exhaustion are part of the mission experience!

My first night going back to the ministry work at our church caused butterflies to stir up my stomach as I felt more like I was entering the lion's den than a safe place amongst friends.

I brought all my goodies from the trip, and

made a tropical tray of fruit for our weekly pot-luck and shared my smile with those who weren't so happy with me.

I prepared my heart, knowing that probably they would not respond to my attempt at "doing good." But I felt complete, knowing I was being obedient to God in loving them. As I had antici-pated, no one cheered or seemed to notice the interesting Indonesian treats. No one said anything to me actually. And it was okay.

God instructed me to do good to those who mistreated me and that was my mission fulfilled. He infused me with grace to be kind to them, and to not open my mouth against them to anyone in the ministry there. I left my vindication with Him who is my teacher and example.

It didn't feel good to still be rejected. But I felt a sense of peace, knowing that I could finish my commitment to that season of ministry with dig-nity and continue to grow into the image of Christ which included suffering at the hands of fellow disciples. It was one of his own disciples that be-trayed him with a kiss; and we are not greater than our Lord. If he suffered, he said we shall suffer too.

FORGIVING GRACE

He taught us to pray:

Our Father, who art in heaven,
Hallowed be thy name.
Thy kingdom come, thy will be done,
On earth as it is in heaven.
Give us this day our daily bread and
Forgive of us our trespasses as we forgive those who
Trespass against us. Lead us not into temptation but
Deliver us from evil......

Forgiving grace. He gave it to us. He will give
you the grace to forgive others.

Humorous Grace

Too Spiritual for My Own Good

"Ohhhhhooowwwooohh!" The sound jolted us out of the room to investigate this ghostly gasp! The hairs on my arms were standing up like soldiers at attention. I could almost feel my pupils dilate as the adrenaline surged through my body!

My fearless leadership as the nurse in charge of the Alzheimer's wing was more like "fear-full" leadership though I tried to appear confident. If Superman used his X-ray vision on me, he would have seen my liver quiver!

With trepidation I peered down the long corridors. It was as quiet as the night before Christmas. Not a creature was stirring, not even our therapy dog, Travis. It was 10:00 a.m., and most of the residents in our assisted living facility memory care unit were taking their "morning naps."

Once again, "OOOOHHHOOWWWWW-OO!" The sound was like a wolf howling at the moon! I scanned the halls again and noted three little women asleep on a loveseat.

To my astonishment this horrendous noise was coming from the vocal cords of 98-year-old Juanita. Juanita's weight was probably the same as her age. She never opened her eyes as she howled, which added to this eeriness of the setting.

Many mornings after breakfast, Juanita, Naomi, and Bernie sat squished together on that loveseat like sardines in a can. Each of these ladies' heads was on the other's shoulder.

Juanita and the other two snoozers appeared undisturbed, though the mournful crier had me and two care givers hyper-alert and unnerved!

Now my astute nursing skills came into action---I looked at Juanita. Her lips were pink. She was breathing and her skin was warm. I deduced that she was not dying and this was always a good thing in my profession!

Next, I did a spiritual assessment. I don't typically do this type of assessment but then again I don't usually have the sound of a *screamin' demon* coming from my patients either. My thoughts raced: "Does she have a demon? Is she possessed? Can it really be possible for a sweet 98-year-old lady to be possessed?" Like Sherlock Holmes, I paced a bit, keeping my eyes on Juanita the whole time.

Again, "OOOOOHHOOOWWWWOOOO-WHH!" howled Juanita!

With authority, though trembling, I stepped up to the loveseat with my hand outstretched and commanded the questionable demon to "Be quiet in Jesus name!" To my own amazement, now I was acting less like Holmes and more like a T.V. preacher.

Puzzled, but respectful, my two staff members stood by my side and just stared at me. I looked at them and thought to myself, "They probably think I am the one who is possessed." I turned my attention back to Juanita and tried not to think about what they were thinking.

The lady in the middle of the loveseat was Naomi. She resembled a figure on a totem pole; arms crossed over her chest, eyes closed and mouth open, poised as stiff as wood. She was so close to Juanita it was as though she were welded onto her.

The mystery of this hair-raising howling ended

as suddenly as it began.

Naomi, still in her totem position, with eyes still closed, tipped ever so slightly to the side and Juanita as if in slow motion, removed her frail purple hand out from under Naomi's behind! The moaning was all over. The case of the screamin' demon was solved. Juanita's hand slowly turned from purple to pink; and all three of the women continued to take their naps—snuggled up against each other.

Now my co-workers and I began howling! We laughed till we hurt and were short of breath! This was definitely a case of "humor in uniform" and I laughed at myself for being "too spiritual for my own good!" I'm glad they gave me grace and I gave myself a second helping too!!!

Painful Grace

"Excuse Me, There is Something in My Eye."

I have this chronic sore spot on my back that I often medicate with an over-the-counter pain cream. This ointment burns and feels good at that same time. It's called "PAIN BUSTER."

I also have a tendency to point out things to my husband that burn or irritate me instead of perhaps praying about it first, or being "gentle" in my speech. I'm more like an Amtrak racing at 70 miles an hour to get my point across. Not a good virtue.

So, one Sunday morning, I was quite annoyed at what I perceived as his lack of spirituality; I zoomed into the bathroom where he was reading a book in the tub. I then snapped out my reasons for why he should go to church. Then, I blasted out of the bathroom and got ready to go "worship."

I huffed out of the house and took my self-righteous self to church, feeling annoyed at having to go alone. Like eating a caramel, I sort of enjoyed chewing on all the things I'd said to him because I thought he deserved it.

When I arrived back at home, I went to our bedroom because I now had a headache and a back-ache (imagine that!) I popped two extra strength Tylenol and got my tube of Pain Buster ointment and rubbed some on my back. Feeling exhausted from my emotional outburst hours earlier, I slunk into bed and curled up in my quilt. With a deep yawn I got ready for a much- needed nap. A knock came at the bedroom door.

"Can we talk?" my husband asked.

I looked at him, or should I say, tried to look at him, because I'd gotten pain killer in one of my eyes, and it was tearing and burning so much that I couldn't open it. I couldn't exactly give him the evil eye at this point; which was probably God's grace considering the damage I'd already done with my tongue!

I agreed, knowing it wasn't going to an easy talk after my morning's escapade. I tried to look at him, but my eye was on fire. Apparently I'd gotten some of the pain cream in it when I rubbed it.

"Excuse me," I said, " I have something in my eye." I got up to wash my hands and went to get some tissues and wash my hands when I realized the words that just came out of my mouth were piercing my own heart. I had something in my eye alright and it was more than pain cream.

I sat down to listen to my husband with an attitude of humility. I held a wet rag against my eye the whole time while he explained how hurt he'd felt by my accusations that morning. I realized that what he said was true and that my words had offended his sensitive nature. All of my picking at him was because of my wrong thinking and self righteous religiousness. I apologized to him with sincere humility to him and asked for forgiveness.

I love the way this passage in Matthew chapter 7 is paraphrased in the Message version of the Bible. "Don't pick on people, jump on their failures, or criticize their faults—unless of course you want the same treatment. That critical spirit has a way of boomeranging. It's easy to see a smudge on your neighbor's face and be oblivious to the ugly sneer on your own. Do you have the nerve to say, "Let me wash your face for you," when your own face is distorted by contempt? It's the whole traveling road show mentality all over again, playing a holier than thou part instead of just living your part. Wipe that ugly sneer off your own face, and you might be fit to offer a washcloth to your neighbor."

The boomerang thing—it's a fact! I got what I dished out. In a strange way it did come back and hit me right in the eye!

God works in mysterious ways. He busted my "holier than thou-ness" with Pain Buster cream! He also has a sense of humor and is very loving….I'm glad he forgave me even before the eyes of my heart were even open to my sin and after my confession too. And I'm glad my husband forgave my harsh words and judgmental behavior.

Father in heaven, please help tame my tongue. Convict of me of the harm my words have done. Change me and cleanse me—wash away my sin. Help me be a wife that will love and understand my husband.

Easter Dinner Grace

A Miracle on Main Street

"Mary, can you help us move this weekend?" asked my friend Yola.

With some trepidation I replied, "Of course we can help you move." Yola was my new friend from work.

My hesitation was that it was going to be on Easter weekend and I had a lot of grocery shopping, baking, and meal preparation to do for *my* family and I was sure it would be a huge inconvenience. Somehow, I would manage *to do it all,* I told myself. Doing it all *myself* was a lifelong trap for me it and I still fall into it more than I like to admit.

This particular holiday I planned to make an atypical Easter dinner instead of the traditional ham, potato salad, and yams we were used to. I discovered a recipe for a unique way to serve sliced ham and turkey, layered with Swiss cheese and spinach. These ingredients would then be baked in the middle of rolled pastry dough. Then the sliced pinwheels made for a great presentation on a decorative serving platter. I couldn't wait to get in my kitchen and begin my food art work!

There was one certain traditional food that I was not going to forfeit making with my atypical meal and that was *"lamb cake."* My mother always made lamb cakes as I was growing up, and now I always make one for my own family. It is basically pound cake batter baked in a lamb form pan. After it's cooled, it is iced with vanilla frosting and finally smothered with snow white flaked coconut. I used black jelly beans for the nose and eyes. Carefully placing a red ribbon around its neck, the lamb would be positioned on a bed of Easter grass and become the center piece for our table.

As a child, I thought lamb cakes were cute. As an adult, I understand that Jesus is the Lamb of God; that he was slain for the forgiveness of sin for all mankind, and for me personally. He was the incarnate sacrificial Passover Lamb. The beautiful lamb cake that would be our centerpiece would be broken, slashed and served after our meal.

Well, the holiday weekend roared in and I charged out the door to go help my friends move. After all, *we* had the truck, and my husband and our teen son had the muscles. I did my share of carrying boxes down the flight of stairs from their quarters to the truck and up three flights to their new apartment.

Upon returning home later that afternoon, my "charge" had expired. Feeling as if I was wearing a bell diver's suit, I slogged into my kitchen to begin my Easter dinner shopping list and prep. My food *art work* was looking more like *hard work*. Before starting my list, I had to unload two bags of food that Yola had sent home with me from her place. They were going out of the country for a month just after the weekend and didn't want it to be wasted.

As I packed her things into my refrigerator, it was as though I was putting a puzzle together. Yola had no way of knowing of my dinner plans so this dinner puzzle was quite surprising. I took out a package of sliced ham, then one of sliced turkey, and in the mix, a package of Swiss cheese! To my absolute astonishment, I pulled out a box of freezer pastry dough, just exactly what I needed to make the dinner from the magazine recipe.

Just then there was a knock on our door. My future daughter-in-law stood in the doorway holding a dish on which sat a beautiful lamb cake!

I knew God was blessing us for helping our friends that day. He laid down his life for his friends; and asks us to do the same for others.

When we sat down to dinner on that extraordinary Easter Sunday, we enjoyed an amazing "grace." The grace of a miracle. Our hearts were filled with gratitude.

Project Gold Cross

Signs of Grace

Some folks labeled my mom's friend, Judy, a certifiable "nut"---especially her husband. I, however, and many others--adored her.

Not long after moving to Arizona, Judy was diagnosed with stage 4 ovarian cancer and needed an extensive operation to save her life. Her small frame melted away like a snow cone on a July day and her strength withered to nothing. But it was here---the desert place of her life---that she met Christ. She felt alone, deserted, in a place of soul-drought.

"You have work to do; I'm not done with you yet." That's what the voice had told her in a vision following her surgery. When Judy gave this testimony at my mom's Bible study group, she was not being a "nut." It was real. She now looked like the picture of health and one would never know the ravaging disease had ever visited her.

Compelled to do work the Lord had told her to do, Judy would openly sing and pray and encourage others all around her. She was like a joy magnet and one couldn't help but be drawn to her. At the nursing home where I worked; she would sing with one person like she was singing with a thousand. She was not a very good singer but joy flowed from her like a river. Not only did she sing badly, she would dance a jig and say "Praise the Lord! Hallelujah!"

One day Judy showed up at my mom's house with a secretive request. She trusted my mother, Marge, with an idea, or may I say a "vision" that she believed God had given her. Judy was in her 60s, my mom---well, late 70s I'll say. These were not young girls with weird notions; but mature women with sincere faith in God.

"I need to make a gold cross," Judy said. "I can see it, but I don't know how to make it. I don't even know why I need it; but God has a reason for it. Can you help me?"

So, Marge questioned Judy: "How big do you

need it? What do you want it made from? Tell me more about this cross."

Judy said, "It needs to be six feet tall, it needs to be portable so I can store it under my bed until I need it."

"Six feet tall?" exclaimed Marge. "Do you want it out of wood, metal or what? I can't make a wooden one. I can, however, sew something."

"Okay, let's sew something!" Judy readily agreed. She was the visionary; Marge was her new project engineer.

"I don't know what I need it for; I just know I need to do this," she insisted.

Next, these two friends went to the fabric store, feeling and searching through the bundles, as if on a treasure hunt for just the right material to make the cross. A shimmering gold satin-like fabric was just perfect, with a royal purple silk for a sash to drape over the arms of the cross. The cardboard bolt spoke "pattern" to Marge. "We'll use the bolt for the arms of the cross." And so the cross started coming together as they brainstormed ideas with one another.

"It needs to be able to be disassembled, Marge, so I can put it under my bed." She was adamant about this feature of the project. Under the cardboard bolt, they decided to use PVC pipe for the cross's skeleton to create a firm-standing cross.

The work began; Marge laid it all out on the living room floor. Her sewing machine hummed as the cloth flew under its needle and the vision became a reality. The cross remained a secret between her and Marge and her Bible study friends.

Judy had another secret but Marge didn't know about this one, nor the women's group. Since I was a nurse, I guess Judy felt comfortable calling me from home one evening with a problem. She said, "I think my finger is broken."

I asked what happened and she told me that her husband had twisted her arm behind her back when dinner was not prepared exactly on time. I told her to meet me at the emergency room. She reluctantly went to the hospital and had X-rays taken. We prayed and talked together in the exam room as we waited for the results. The films revealed that she did indeed have a fracture and she was informed by the physician that a police officer would be coming to the hospital to take her report. "In Arizona, when someone receives a fractured bone in a domestic dispute, we need to arrest the person who did it," the officer explained. Her husband's abusive behavior was no longer a secret; consequently he spent the night in jail.

Project gold cross was finished. It was assembled and then finally disassembled to be placed in storage under Judy's bed; just as she saw in the vision. It was buried in darkness; like a flower bulb in the fall, buried in the dirt and covered up to protect it during the winter months.

The winter season of life now stormed in on Judy once again. She began feeling weak and lost her appetite. She continued to make her daily visits to the nursing home where she ministered to the elderly. Her picture of health was changing into the image of a person with a grave illness. Her weight again melted away; her color turned to a pasty gray. She became bed-bound in a matter of weeks. The cancer was back.

My last visit with Judy was at the hospital. She lay in her hospital bed with rosary beads in her hand and a large nasal-gastric tube in her nose and throat. I held her bony hand in mine and in a hoarse voice she said, "I want to pray for you."

"Pray for me?" I was aghast. *"I should be praying for her, not the other way around."* Her humility accosted me. We had prayed together many times before and so we did again. After praying, I kissed her cool, frail hand. It was a bittersweet visit. She died two days later.

"We're going to go get the cross, MaryBeth. Come and pick me up!" my mom commanded over the phone. I wasn't sure about this new mission. I wasn't feeling the courage to go to Judy's house and ask her husband if we could look under the bed for the cross.

"We're gonna put it up in her yard!" mom barked like General Patton!

She called Judy's husband and, to our surprise, he was quite compliant regarding the idea of erecting the gold cross.

After finding and assembling the cross, we looked for a place to erect it. There was a place just waiting for it. It happened to be in the center of their front yard which was located on a busy corner of their neighborhood. Many who lived there knew Judy personally and had attended neighborhood prayer gatherings with her more than once.

A giant saguaro stood staring at us. It was very tall and straight. We positioned the cross carefully so we wouldn't pierce ourselves with the needle-sharp thorns. It was very windy this day, however, and the cross needed more support, so we tied it against the cactus. Its thorns hugged the cross to its side. As I examined the nail-like spikes on the cactus, I couldn't help but think how painful the thorny crown was that they forced on Jesus' head.

The sun was beginning to set as we pulled away from Judy's home. Its blinding rays focused directly on the golden cross and it appeared ablaze. Someone drove by and honked. It felt like a standing ovation! The royal purple banner flowed wildly as the wind lifted it up and about. It was a beautiful sight to behold.

I didn't remember until we were driving away that the next day was Easter Sunday. When I did realize it, the joy of the Lord swelled in my heart. Judy was with Jesus now. He said, "I am the Resurrection and the Life, He who believes in me shall never die."

Project gold cross is a picture that is forever etched in my mind; I will never forget its story.

Grace for Those in the Dark

**Though I Sit in the Darkness,
The Lord is my Light.**

Friend and co-worker, Dr. Steve Anderson reported that he typically saw about one bilaterally blind person per year in his Minneapolis practice. In contrast, on a month-long mission trip to West Kalimantan this past June, we saw many bilaterally blind people each day. .

Blindness from cataracts is one of the only curable types of blindness and intervention is crucial in developing nations of the world such as Indonesia. Barring any other pathology such as glaucoma, diabetic retinopathy, or retinal detachment, a thirty-minute procedure performed by an ophthalmologist can return sight to a person who is blind from cataracts. The procedure is surgically removing the opaque lens, called a cataract, and replacing it with a synthetic intraocular lens into the lens capsule. Often no sutures are required though occasionally a few are put in, depending on the surgeon's technique and the patient's need.

My experience as a nurse and an ophthalmic assistant has allowed me to see first-hand in the United States, Honduras, and Indonesia, the stark differences in medical care and its availability; and I am a changed person for it. People are the same all over the world. We all experience pain, loss, fear, and need, in the same manner. We all desire wellness and hope for our loved ones. When there is no hope, there is great sadness and grief. Being a short term missionary and bringing the gift of sight to the hopeless has opened the eyes of my heart. My vision is to continue to bring hope to the poverty stricken blind.

Recently I learned that the population of Borneo is approximately twenty-four million; and there are five ophthalmologists on the entire island. I was astounded. I personally know five ophthalmologists that have offices less than five miles from where I live, and the population of the surrounding towns is less than 50,000. To realize that so many people would possibly never have an opportunity for eye care was more than I could comprehend.

On my most recent trip to help establish a new eye clinic at a village hospital, I was again reminded of the great need for eye health care. On one of our patient screening days, we encountered a thirty-six-year-old man who had been bilaterally blind for two years. He was led into our exam room by his wife; he could not identify the chair or direction which it faced. His intraocular pressures were 45 in each eye (normal being less than 20), which gave us an indication that, even though we could remove his cataracts, he may not achieve normal vision. The doctor was unable to view the back of the eye to see if there was any optic nerve damage due to the fact the patient also had extremely tiny, fixed pupils secondary to posterior synechiae (that is, the iris was stuck to the surface of the lens) as well as dense cataracts. As the doctor explained the possibility of a poor outcome, the man's wife wept. My heart felt as though it were breaking with hers. She had come with so much hope for help; and the idea of her husband having no sight was overwhelming to her.

Later that day, I asked them if I could pray for

them before they left. She could only nod as the tears kept her from speaking. We held hands and called on the name of Jesus, remembering that all things are possible with God.

We saw several patients with huge, fixed pupils, indicating glaucoma or some other pathology causing blindness that could probably not be improved with surgery, whether they had cataracts or not. Unfortunately for these patients, we were unable to offer them any hope.

As an ophthalmic assistant for many years, I have been trained to assess pupils, anterior chamber depths, and to take intraocular pressures. I screened many patients in Indonesia with narrow anterior chambers, high pressure and decreased vision because of the glaucoma disease process. In America, when people come in for routine eye exams, these things are always assessed and if a patient is what we call a "glaucoma suspect," they are treated with eye drops or sometimes they receive treatment with a laser to put a hole in the iris to allow intraocular pressure to remain low. This is called an iridectomy. If a patient has untreated glaucoma, blindness is an irreversible certainty.

Prior to their session with the eye doctor, I saw a very common pattern with these particular patients when I took their history. Commonly, they reported: "At first I had pain in my eye (or eyes); then the pain went away, and now I cannot see." This indicated to me that, specifically with narrow angle glaucoma, the pain they experienced at first was from high intraocular pressure. Because they were not treated, the pressure caused damage on the back of the eye at the optic nerve, resulting in vision loss over a period of time. The amount of damage to the optic nerve depended on how high the pressure was and how long the problem had remained. Their physical assessments when we examined them many months or years after they first sensed "pain" showed large, fixed 8-9mm pupils and their visual acuities indicated obvious vision loss. Any patient that complains of eye pain should always be assessed for high intraocular pressure.

In America, the patients I have seen with acute narrow-angle glaucoma are in obvious pain and many of them experience nausea and vomiting. It is considered a medical emergency like heart attack or stroke. Without intervention, the patient loses the vision in the affected eye.

We saw a number of patients with dense cataracts as well as macular scars. We performed cataract surgery on them, only to find out after the surgery that macular scarring was present. The pupils on these patients don't usually give any sign of this type of eye problem. Again, the doctor cannot see into the back of the eye just as the patient cannot see out of the eye because of the dense opacity. Though some still have a macular problem and can't see straight ahead to read or drive a vehicle, they do appreciate marginally better peripheral vision, and can get around better in the daily activities of life.

We had the great privilege of seeing our surgical patients post-operatively both on day one and week one. Many of them had much-improved vision without the need for spectacle correction. Those that did not improve were those who had some added pathology. Regarding the thirty-six-year-old man I mentioned previously, we performed cataract surgery on both of his eyes. He was able to walk into the exam room alone, not being led around by his wife. Unlike the first time he came to our clinic, his countenance was bright, he held his head up and appeared smiling and confident. His wife was also smiling. He could count fingers, which is not particularly good vision; but enough to be able to ambulate independently and move about freely. He was able to find the exam chair and to seat himself. That morning in my personal devotions I'd read from Psalm 146:8 "The Lord gives sight to the blind." Puji Tuhan! Actually, that's exactly what this patient said to us, "Puji Tuhan" (translation: Praise the Lord!)

Bringing the gift of sight physically to the people of West Kalimantan was a great blessing to me. Bringing the good news of the Gospel of Jesus Christ was also a great blessing. At the end of our one day post op checks we would gather our patients and their family members and express our appreciation to them for letting us serve them. I would tell them how the god of this world, Satan, has blinded the minds and hearts of people lest they should see and believe on the one true God and his Son, Jesus Christ. Then I prayed that God would open the eyes of their hearts to believe for the forgiveness of their sins, and to receive God's great love for them. My cup overflowed.

To those that were irreversibly blind, I reminded them of the passage from Isaiah 50:10, "Let him who walks in the dark, who has no light, trust in the name of the Lord and rely on his God." And to this I say, "Puji Tuhan."

I mused in silence about my time in West Kalimantan, and the love I felt for our patients and new brothers and sisters in Christ. I came across another scripture that expressed the thoughts of my heart. The apostle, Paul, says it all here in Ephesians chapter 1 verses 15-19; "For this reason, ever since I heard about your faith in the Lord Jesus and your love for all the saints, I have not stopped giving thanks for you, remembering you in my prayers. I keep asking the God of our Lord Jesus Christ, the glorious Father, may give you the Spirit of wisdom, and revelations, so that you may know him better. I pray also that eyes of your heart may be enlightened in order that you may know the hope to which he has called you, the riches of his inheritance in the saints, and his incomparably great power for us who believe."

I look forward with much anticipation to returning again to our newborn eye clinic and being with dedicated believers, physicians, nurses and friends from Indonesia and other parts of the world, as we bring the gift of sight to the blind.

Even Dogs Need Grace

Dog Day Afternoon

It was a dog day afternoon this past Father's Day. My husband and I seemed strangely quiet this particular morning. We are empty nesters.

My husband had come home from work the day before and exuberantly spoke about the irresistible red pup he saw on television. The local channel was airing a story at a local animal shelter and inviting people to come and adopt one of their canine residents.

"What do you think?" he asked. We'd already been tossing the idea around for months. I was reluctant about the puppy idea because of all the adjustments that come with any baby!

We decided to go look at the local pound after church. Still the quietness between us felt odd. Both of us were missing our grown son, but didn't voice the feelings of longing for him. It was just the two of us now.

Arriving at the first animal shelter, we ventured in to see if the adorable pup was still there. We passed cage after cage. Some barked, some growled and showed sharp teeth, while others curled up in the corners of their fenced kennels. But no red pup.

"It was taken right away," the volunteer said. "But there is another place you might look though."

With instructions in hand, we headed out to look at more dogs.

"What are we doing?" I asked myself. *"Is this a good idea?"* We hadn't had a pet for several years. We also had moved several times.

"Sometimes I wish our lives were more stable," I said to my husband. "We have moved so much. I desire more stability in our lives."

The new city animal shelter was quite impressive. A beautiful prayer framed the welcoming doors to the facility. It read:

FOR BIRDS WITH BROKEN WINGS,
FOR RABBITS CAUGHT IN SPRINGS,
FOR POOR BEWILDERED FOXES,

EVEN DOGS NEED GRACE

AND BUTTERFLIES IN BOXES,
FOR DOGS WITHOUT A HOME,
FOR CATS THAT WALK ALONE,
FOR HORSES WORN AND OLD,
FOR SHEEP WITHOUT A FOLD,
FOR ALL THOSE WEAK AND LONELY,
AND DEPENDING ON MAN SOLEY,
BY ALL WE HOLD MOST HOLY,
HEAR US WE BESEECH THEE OH LORD.

This prayer captured my heart. I began to think this was a good idea, after all.

So, again we traipsed by the barking, growling, jumping dogs in one kennel after the next. Every size, shape, color and breed seemed to be represented. Amidst the noise and activity of the curious creatures lay one golden retriever, looking oddly calm. We stopped and looked at her. The name tag on the kennel read "Angel." It appeared she was as gentle and loving as an angel. "Is she ill?" I wondered. She was so calm compared to the jumpers and barkers all around her.

We had the volunteer bring her out to see us. We went in a small room with her to see her more intimately. She cowered and came to us to be petted. She trembled nervously as we inspected her. Her face was irresistible, and her golden color was strikingly attractive. We both liked her almost instantly.

Having viewed the rest of the dogs, we were drawn again to Angel's kennel. After talking it over, I said, "Let's pray. God will show us if we should take her." The next step was to speak with a dog adoption counselor.

We had to take a quick test to see if we "qualified" to be pet owners.

After answering the many questions, and adding up our score, we turned the page over to see if our score qualified us. To our delight it read, "Congratulations, you appear to be a STABLE family and are now ready to be a pet owner!" Here was our confirmation!

With a new red leash and collar, we brought Angel home. Our home now was filled with a little more activity, but still quiet! I wondered if our new dog had the ability to bark or not. We didn't hear a squeak out of her. Finally, when the lawn maintenance man came by, we discovered she definitely had a bark. And a loud one at that! She was a protector for sure.

Angel is a joy and a comfort to me and my family. I know that God cares for his creatures, every one. Take a dog day afternoon and go check out your local animal shelter. You might want to take some cash; and say a prayer. Maybe God wants to bless you with an "Angel" too....

Even dogs need grace---a loving home---and someone to care for them. God loves all his creatures great and small...

Behind Closed Doors

Grace Required.

So, what does go on behind closed doors? Where I work, it's the care of 17 senior adults with dementia or Alzheimer's Disease.

Daily living needs are met, food is served, activities are coordinated, and beds are made ready for these residents in our assisted living facility. What else goes on behind closed doors in memory care units such as ours? Here's the nitty gritty for enquiring minds who want to know. Some residents are lonely. They have outlived their family members. Friends at their age are few, it appears.

Some pace up and down the halls, up and down the halls... Our doors are secured so they can't get lost. Behind those doors are folks just like you and me. Perhaps they would remind you of your family members, or maybe one of them is your family member.

Many of them don't remember what they had for lunch; but they can recite the Lord's Prayer by heart from past memory. They don't know the latest tunes, but their eyes sparkle, some from tears, as they sing the hymns that we all love and know. The doxology is also imprinted in the deep recesses of their minds....

Though a large hall calendar keeps track of the date, days merge into each other in this place. Several residents can still remember a time in their life when God touched their hearts. Recently one woman testified of sensing God's presence at summer camp as a child. Another resident stated that his mother would often make him pray with her outside the house after he spent a night of carousing with his friends! Another woman said, "My mother always prayed with us; she was always kind and never raised her voice at us."

As we look to God's Word for hope and help, let us encourage those who can no longer read the words on pages or understand them. These same people understand human touch, a smile, an uplifting word just like you and I do.

BEHIND CLOSED DOORS

James 1:27 declares, "Religion that God our Father accepts as pure and faultless is this; to look after orphans and WIDOWS IN THEIR DISTRESS, and to keep oneself pure from being polluted by the world." On my unit, we have many widows with memory problems who are often distressed.

As Christians, the opportunity to minister to widows is all around us. A vast mission field to work in is right here in our backyards.

Having personally done Sunday morning outreach services for this group of people with memory troubles has enlightened me probably more than them! I have seen the hearts of these dear people.

Their minds and memory may not be what they used to be; but their hearts are still touched by the presence of God. I've observed some with tear-filled eyes and faces full of adoration as they sang hymns. Some have even raised their hands unashamedly in praise to Him! Their hearts have not forgotten the love of God or the presence of the Holy Spirit.

Sometimes I wonder if it is us Christians who are the ones with a memory problem. Do we re-member the command to "GO-- ye into ALL the world"? We have trouble just going to our back-yard to minister to people, much less ALL the world!

Behind the closed doors of nursing homes and memory care facilities; few people come to visit. Behind closed doors are fine senior men and women with mental afflictions who suffer the loneliness that shut ins do. One woman repeats over and over, "I'm all alone, I'm all alone now, all alone..."

May we not be comfortable behind the doors of our churches, our small group gatherings or our homes. Instead, may our hearts be stirred to remember the poor, the afflicted, the widows and orphans as Jesus did. He sees exactly "what goes on behind closed doors."

Some things to do while visiting a nursing home:

- *Bring a few stuffed animals*
- *Smile at the people*
- *Just hold someone's hand*
- *Share a bag of Tootsie Pop suckers (they can't choke on a sucker; ask the nurses first!)*
- *Call ahead to see if you can bring your own dog to visit; I do this and it's a hit!*

BEHIND CLOSED DOORS

- *Bring a small child with you or a few--(the elderly love to see children)*
- *Read a story to somebody*
- *Share some photographs of theirs or yours with them*

Gracious Care Giver

Annie

She sashayed down the hall of the nursing home like a ghost in her over-sized cloak. Her head was smothered by a "babushka" that hid her delicate features. A frail figure was buried beneath the bulky trench coat. Black boots silently transported her to her friend who was seated in the hall in a wheelchair.

She spoke some words and handed a Christmas poinsettia to her friend. I overheard the gentle visitor speak and my head turned as though I'd heard a favorite song. I knew this song; but how? I listened and stared at the fragile lady in the trench coat and boots.

"Could it possibly be?" I mused. *"How old could she*

be now? Could it really be her?" My heart knew from the first sounds of her voice that it was indeed Annie. It was Annie!

Annie was a nurse's aide that I met in 1978. Do the math: 28 years earlier. She took care of my father during the last weeks of his life. She also took care of my husband when he almost lost a finger in a work accident and another time when he was critically ill.

Even back then she was thin; and what I considered "old" to be working so hard. She always smiled, and never appeared to be bothered if patients needed something or if a nurse asked her to do something. She was gentle and kind and never in a hurry.

I couldn't resist asking her, "Are you Annie?"

"Yes," she said and looked at me without recognition. I told her how I knew her; but, of course, she didn't remember me or my family. She had taken care of hundreds of people in her time; and it looked as though she still was. I recognized the smile, the soft voice, and the kindness.

I asked her if I could give her a hug. We embraced; I felt her bony frame through the coat.

When I spoke her name aloud, other nurses and people in the hall also recognized her. They began sharing their stories of knowing her and their responses were just like mine. Hugs, smiles and warm fuzzies filled the air like snowflakes on a wintry day.

I hope I will always remember my encounter with this dear woman. She is obviously not "re-tired" in her work for the Lord. I heard her talk about friends from the "church" and her ministry continues at the ripe old age of____;---well, I don't know; but it reminds me that I want to emulate the kindness and gentleness she exudes.

I've heard it said, ""People die as they have lived," and elderly, gracious Annie, inspires me to be thinking more and more about how to live.

My Dash?

"What will you do with your dash?" my 81-year-old mother asked me. She was sharing with me an inspiring sermon she'd recently heard and I needed the encouragement as I was preparing to go to Indonesia on a mission trip with Vision Outreach International.

You have to know a little about me to appreciate the need for encouragement. My nickname as a kid was "Scary Mary." I was scared of everything. I was scared to go to kindergarten and cried every day for the first week. My teacher sat me behind the walk in play house with a dunce cap on for crying. I learned to be ashamed of being afraid.

My sister Nora and I used to drink a pretend drink when we were very young. We called it "lemon-fraid." It was a drink that would help us to not be afraid! We'd laugh as we drank our super duper drink! Kids do weird things.

Not being a kid anymore, I still had fears eating at my insides like termites on a log pile. Indonesia was the furthest I'd ever been away from any of my family members. Also, though I'd flown plenty of times before this opportunity, I still wasn't too fond of flying.

"What will you do with your dash?" She went on to explain: "The dash is literally the dash on your tombstone. You know, the date you were born comes first, then the dash, then the date of your death. The dash represents what you do with your life between your birth and your death. Go for it! God will be with you; don't be afraid."

"Only one life will soon be past. Only what's done for Christ will last." This is a quote I've heard many times and believe to be true. All other worldly pursuits are empty and do not last. I know I want my life—my dash—in this world to last eternally.

As I ponder the idea of the dash, tombstones, and life; I recall a walk I took in the cemetery where my father is buried. As I walked I'd look at tombstones and read the epitaphs. Oddly, my first missionary assignment was in my own hometown to an elderly man whose headstone ended up right across from my father's gravesite.

I wanted to be a missionary. God sent me to

this old gentleman who lived on a farm and was wheelchair bound. He had rheumatoid (crippling) arthritis and needed help with bathing, foot care and shampooing his nearly hairless head. He also needed companionship, conversation and some TLC. During each visit, we would talk and share Hardees' sausage biscuits and coffee. He especially liked the cinnamon rolls. I like that his gravesite is right near my father's. That way, I will never forget him.

Just down a bit further is a headstone that has these words engraved on it. ***"The eyes of the Lord search to and fro throughout the earth, searching for a man whose heart is fully committed to Him,"*** II Chron. 16:9.

Then I read the name on the gravestone and realized who it was. It was the man who started Life Action Ministry many years ago. "He was so young," I thought. And yet his dash in my mind is soooo big.

I am still working on my dash. Whether it's visiting someone in a nursing home, dancing with my granddaughter or going overseas on medical mission trips; I want my dash to count. Now I can ask you--what will you do with your dash?

Pool Infused Grace

Invisible Doors

The meteorologist said it could be "near-freezing temperatures" in Phoenix tonight, so I thought it would be a good idea to bring my potted flowers indoors overnight. My porch is sweetly decorated with a lovely wooden bench, a hummingbird feeder, hanging wind chimes and a colorful windsock.

Picking up my pots packed with pansies, I turned and promptly crashed right into the sliding glass door! Wham! My nose and forehead left a make-up smear on the glass after bouncing off the door! My body stung with pain from my forceful encounter with the colorless barrier!

There on the couch sat my husband, observing the whole thing. He just sat there, expressionless.

As I opened the door, we looked at one another and burst into hilarious laughter!

We continued to laugh so much that tears ran down my face, my nose ran like a faucet, and audible wheezing left me gasping for air!

A few moments later I could breathe well enough to share a few words of wisdom. "When God closes a door, don't try to walk through it!" And we laughed some more.

As funny as this incident was to me a few months ago, it doesn't seem as funny to me today. I have had the experience of running into invisible doors many times over the last few months.

After many tears and prayers, I gave my notice at work. It was a hostile work environment and I am a peacemaker. I did not understand why this had to happen at this time in my life. It weighed heavily on my heart. We had just moved recently to Arizona and were anticipating new beginnings that were fresh and exciting. But it seemed as though my excitement was now turning to discouragement.

This incident didn't take me by total surprise, however. I felt a familiar sense of déjà vu. Though the circumstances were different now, the act of having to wait on the Lord for his help was what would be needed to get through the coming weeks and perhaps months ahead.

Knowing this in my heart and living it out in my life became my work. I became totally occupied with the word of God and waiting in silence to hear his voice.

On my very first day home from the job, I went swimming in our courtyard pool. Swimming back and forth like an athlete in training, I tried to wear down my panic and fear of the future. After much exertion, it struck me that all of my own energy and strength is not what God wanted. He didn't need my efforts or strength to take care of my future.

In a still small voice, I heard, "Stand still." The voice came again. "What do you see? All I saw were my feet in the bottom of the pool and a little debris floating at the bottom. Then suddenly, it was there. To my right on the surface of the water: the reflection of three palm trees. My Bible reading that morning confirmed the sight on the water. Psalm 92:12 says, "The righteous shall flourish like a palm tree."

Pondering the verse and the reflection of the palms gave me a renewed sense of hope. Palm trees stand very tall and can take days and months of intense heat year after year. Yet they remain green and bend with the wind whether it is gentle or violent. I felt God was saying to me, that despite the intense heat of my trial, I *would flourish like the palm*. Flourish defined by Webster's means to grow vigorously, to thrive and be at the peak of development. Wow! The situation was looking much different, viewing it through the word of God. My perspective and attitude were changed by this moment of "standing still."

There is another example in the book of Exodus where Moses told the Israelites, "Do not be afraid. Stand firm and you will see the deliverance the Lord will bring you today. The Lord will fight for you; you need only to be still." He told them this as the vast Egyptian army was closing in on them. They had nowhere to run because the Red Sea was before them. They were surrounded. Their situation appeared hopeless. Then the miracle. The Red Sea parted as Moses stretched out his hand over the sea and the Lord drove the waters back with a powerful east wind. I would say he opened the door of the sea.

I had tried to apply for several jobs over a period of months only to crash into more invisible doors. It was painful and humiliating. Just like the time when I and my flower pots crashed into the sliding glass door. My fears felt like an army of en-emies surrounding me and closing in on me. *How can we continue to meet our financial needs without my pay-check? What about our future? What about our savings account?* I fretted.

Psalm 37:7 reminds also, "Be still before the Lord and wait patiently for him." It's not my nature to "be still" or "patient." I want to do something! Fix it. Make it work. Plan my work and work my plan! Being still is still uncomfortable for me!

I know that God's ways are higher than my ways; so I will choose to "be still, and wait for him." I am reminded of an old song I learned when I was 16. It goes like this:

Be ye still; and know that I am God….Be ye still; and filled up with my peace…Be ye still…and know that I am the Lord….and be comforted in me…

I will call you to be lowly; there's a cross you'll have to bear; you must leave the world behind you; and the burden we will share….

I am glad that God promises that anyone who waits for him will not be disappointed. If you are running into closed doors in your life; wait for the Lord; and he will not disappoint you…. Let God's word infuse your mind, calm your heart, and hold you while you wait upon Him.

Painful Grace

Pain Before Healing

On a medical mission trip last year to a jungle village, I was again a member of the "eye team" and our goal was to perform cataract surgery on those blind from cataracts. I have observed this surgery many times in the United States. But, needless to say, performing this procedure is much different in a jungle mission compound hospital.

My assigned duty on this mission was to give the patients the local anesthetic to numb the eye so the patient would not feel the surgery, and to keep the eye from moving. In America, medical doctors often perform this local anesthetic block after the patient is sedated because it is very uncomfortable.

GRACE INFUSIONS

Well, my coworker and brother in Christ, Dr. David Brown taught me the basics of administering this block while in flight to Borneo. I asked many questions, but the whole idea made me feel queasy. In the medical profession we often use this phrase when training others to do a procedure, "See one, teach one, do one." And that's just what happened for me. I saw Dr. David administer this deep injection under the eye, with 5cc of medication that burns. Then, it was my turn. And the next 69 people were mine to do.

The first day we began our surgeries, I was sweating profusely from the 100 degree temperatures. The humidity was also sky-high, as we were right on the equator off the coast of the South China Sea. As I gave the first few painful injections under the patients' eyes, I perspired even more. My neck muscles were tensed, and my face felt tight as I inflicted this awful anesthetic block to these people who so wanted to see again.

Some of them cried out, "Sockeed, sockeed!!" This means, "Pain, painful! Sick!" However, I had no choice but to deliver the painful block so they could proceed with the surgery. I agonized silently as I inserted each inch-and-a-half-long needle below the orbit of their eye. Most were stoic and endured silently, but some were not. After one woman cried out in distress, I glared at my mission team mate, Tom, and voiced my agony: "I can't do this one more time."

He looked at me intently and said words that ring in my ears yet today. He calmly instructed me, "Sister, there must be pain before healing."

I knew it was the truth. I had to continue to cause them momentary pain for them to be able to see again for the rest of their lives. I am a merciful person. I don't like to hurt anyone. But I knew in my heart I must be brave and strong, and do the procedure to each and every one of them. I prayed, "Jesus, help me. Jesus, please help me."

And He did. I grew more confident each time I gave one of the anesthetic blocks.

This is such a picture in my own mind of how God allows pain in our lives; before He can heal us. Pain causes us to evaluate: 1) how we are living 2) our relationship with Him, and 3) how we are treating those around us. It actually can help us see more clearly.

The truth of God's Word is often painful as it pierces our hearts and reveals sin in our lives. Heb. 4:12, "For the Word of God is living, and active. Sharper than any double –edged sword, it penetrates even to dividing soul and spirit, joints and marrow; it judges the thoughts and attitudes of the heart."

As a Christian I find now as I tell others the gospel of Jesus Christ I am afraid at first to cause anyone pain as I speak the truth. But the more I do it, the braver and stronger I become, just as in giving the painful injections I described. I know now, with the Word of God, I must let the truth pierce other's hearts as it has pierced my own at times, and let God heal and restore the hearer. If I do not speak the truth of the gospel, it would be like me refusing to give the anesthetic to the blind patient. They would never be able to have the surgery and receive their sight.

I heard a prominent radio pastor say, "I know God has called me to comfort the afflicted, and also to afflict the comforted." I love this quote. I find it easy as a Christian to comfort the afflicted too, but I am learning to let the Holy Spirit speak or work through me to afflict the comforted, or the comfortable, as I testify of Him and His Word to them.

The truth is that we are all blind and in the dark until we accept the sacrifice of Jesus' death and resurrection for our sins. Jesus suffered excruciating pain for us so we could receive healing for our incurable disease called, "sin." We remain blind until we accept his painful grace; his death on the cross.

Pain before healing. Do you want to be healed? Do you want to see clearly?

Grace for the Blind

Miraculous Restoration

Meridan, age 39, had been blind for 10 years when we met him.

He had a mature cataract in his right eye, and the lens in his left eye had fallen back into the vitreous many years before this exam.

Dr. Steve Anderson performed a cataract extraction surgery on the right eye and we patched it, then sent him to the patient ward. We would see him in the morning for a post op check.

That evening I felt compelled to walk down to the village hospital on the mission compound to visit our patients seen that day. The nurses at the nurse station giggled when I showed up. I wondered if it was something I was wearing, or how

I appeared. I know my size alone probably made them laugh as I am *"very healthy"* according to one of our blind patients who had felt my upper arms. This village is made up of Dayak people, a native tribe of that area of Borneo. Most women there reached only my shoulder in height and I am 5' 4. Their clothing size is probably 0-6, and probably a 14 in girls' sizes for adult women. And no, I'm not divulging what my size is!

Anyway, they continued to giggle and tried to convey a message to me to come and see something in a patient's room. I got the message from their gestures that perhaps there was a mouse in this room. With trepidation and curiosity, I followed them.

They opened the door to the patient's room and there it was. A poster of Mickey Mouse mounted on the stark white hospital wall. They were so pleased and happy to show it to me. Of course I giggled with them too. And then I saw Meridan lying right below the poster.

He wasn't smiling or giggling with the young nurses as they conversed in their native tongue back and forth about Mickey Mouse. He lay there; expressionless, in the dark---even with the large fluorescent light on above him. His surgical eye patched, and blind in the other.

I touched his hand, and said a few things that I know he couldn't understand because of the language barrier; but I believe he understood my body language.

The next morning we removed his patch and he beamed. He had almost 20/30 vision and could see his wife's face, those around him, and even Mickey. His vision was miraculously restored. You have to know, on the island of Borneo, with 24 million people, and only five ophthalmologists, it was a miracle for this young man to receive his sight back.

He was so happy he shed tears. We talked some more and he said to me, "Can I call you my sister?" and I readily replied with much joy, "Yes, and **you are my brother.**"

He Ain't Heavy, He's my Brother

The road is long, with many a winding turn, that leads us to who, knows where, who knows where.
But I'm strong, strong enough to carry him,
He ain't heavy, he's my brother…..
So, on we go-- his welfare is my concern. No burden is he, to bear, we'll get there.

GRACE INFUSIONS

For I know, he would not encumber me, He ain't heavy,
he's my brother
If I'm laiden, at all, I'm laden, with sadness; that ev-
eryone's heart isn't filled with the gladness,
Of love, for one another
It's a long, long road, from which there is no return—
While we're on the way, to there; Why not share? And
the load, doesn't weigh me down at all—He ain't heavy,
he's my brother......

Lyrics by Bobby Scott and Bob Russell

Merciful Grace

The Man with the Towel

I watched him slink toward the old metal folding chair facing the doctor. *What was going on?* We were screening patients for our cataract surgery schedule. The potential candidates were packed in the room like sardines to see the American doctor.

Those who were waiting in line started backing away, covering their noses and mouths with their hands or hankies as the man with a towel approached the chair. A grimy old towel draped over his bowed head masked his disease, but his shame was out in the open for all to view. A foul odor permeated the small exam room. He unveiled his head and gazed at the American doctor with hopeful expectation.

"I'm sorry. There is nothing I can do," the physician stated with sadness in his eyes.

The tumor protruding from the man's eye had also invaded half of his face. His countenance plunged like the Titanic into bleak emptiness. My heart sank, too, as I heard the words, "..nothing I can do."

This moment is forever etched in my memories. The people covering their mouths and backing away--the man's hopes dashed in an instant. It reminded me of examples in the Bible of how lepers were treated. They were kept "outside" society to live with their diseased bodies and broken lives. They were considered *unclean and hopeless*. The shame of being unclean must have been as bad or worse than the disease itself.

That morning's devotional was ringing in my ears as I sat in disbelief, staring at this unfortunate man with the inoperable tumor. "The kingdom of heaven is near. Heal the sick, raise the dead, cleanse those who have leprosy, drive out demons. Freely you have received, freely give." Matthew 10:8 NIV.

Before opening our clinic that day, we three missionaries ate breakfast together, prayed, sang hymns and shared God's word. I told them that

I thanked God for my nursing skills, but as a Christian I felt the need to also pray for people the way the scriptures instructed us too. Little did I know the opportunity would come only hours later.

But would I take the opportunity? Would I pray for a Muslim man in a room packed with people or would I ignore his desperate need? Would my companions think I was a radical weirdo or a Jesus freak if I did? Would I let this suffering individual walk away with no hope--no touch ---no love--nothing?

He lowered his head and swathed the towel over it once again as he prepared to give his seat to the next patient. I looked at my friend Dr. David and asked, "May I pray for this man?" He asked one of our interpreters to ask the Muslim if it would be all right and he welcomed the invitation.

Bowing his head in reverence, he again removed the towel. I came close to him and laid my hand upon his warm moist head and began praying. "In the name of the Father, the Son, and the Holy Spirit." Something was happening; not only to him but in the jam packed exam area. All those near us were bowing their heads and a silence fell over the room. Tears streamed down this man's disfigured face as I prayed. After praying I embraced him gently and he replied in a most broken voice, "Tank you." The cultural and religious barriers were broken and God's love rushed through to him. Many of us near by witnessed God's power.

There was another man with a towel. His name was Jesus. The Holy Son of God used a towel to wash the dirty feet of his disciples and instructed them by saying, "Now that I, your Lord and Teacher have washed your feet, you also should wash one another's feet. I have set you an example that you should do as I have done for you. I tell you the truth; no servant is greater than his master, nor is a messenger greater than the one who sent him. Now that you know these things, you will be blessed if you do them." John 13: 14-15 NIV.

Truth be known, we are all unclean and all of our righteousness is as filthy rags. Jesus washed us clean by his death and resurrection. He laid down his life for us while we were yet his enemies. He reminds us; "Love one another as I have loved you. By this all men will know you that you are my disciples, if you love one another." John 13:34

There aren't many people around us with leprosy or protruding tumor but there are those with drug addictions, sexual sin, mental afflictions and things that cause even us *Christians* to cover our self righteous noses and back away.

Jesus touched the unclean. But will we? Jesus prayed in public for the woman caught in the act of adultery–but would we? He even drew a circle around himself standing right next to the sin-stained woman.

When was the last time you were that close to someone so marked with sin? Would you stand with them during a hard time? Would you befriend them? Would you encourage them?

How about those in prison? Would you visit them? Those with AIDS, would you care for them?

The man with the towel. Have you seen him?

Grace to Wait

Hate to Wait -- Part One

I don't know about you—but *I hate to wait.*

I experienced chronic pain for over six years; and received prayer many times for the same problem. I was waiting for healing. *Waiting…waiting.*

Last November the answer to those prayers became real through the hands of a surgeon. Before my surgery; I remember one particular day on my bed. I was in much distress and agony with the familiar pain. My husband and a friend of ours came into the room; and prayed *again* for me. I felt I couldn't bear it anymore. I had been examined by a new doctor but hadn't heard from him about a surgical date. Soon after my husband finished praying for me; the phone rang. Talk about "answered prayer!"

It was the surgery scheduler from the doctor's office. "How does next month sound?" she asked.

Next month! My heart sank. "That'll be great," I replied, even though it wasn't really true. Once again I had to endure more *waiting*.

Finally the day of surgery arrived. My scheduled time was 4:00 p.m.. I had to wait all day, which gave me time to try not to be nervous, hungry and thirsty! Attempting to remain emotionally calm before major surgery is very difficult, even with many prayers. I felt extremely anxious.

I held tightly to Isaiah 40:29; "He gives strength to the weary and increases the power of the weak" and "those who wait upon the Lord will renew their strength." This helped to anchor my soul as pre-op anxiety tossed me on the ocean of emotion during the wait. I thought of valium too--and how I wished I'd been offered some.

Laying on the gurney with surgical stockings on and an IV line intact ready to be used at 3:00 p.m.: I watched the minutes tick to 4:00 p.m., 4:15, 4:30. Still no sign of the surgeon. *Waiting and more waiting. I hate to wait!*

Finally he arrived. I was rolled off to the O.R. in a flash and onto a stainless steel table; I awakened after the procedure in much pain. Now I would need to *wait* to recover. Hours turned into days; days into weeks. The doctor informed me prior to the procedure that the normal recovery time was six to eight weeks. But three *months* later I discovered that healing has its own time. I had to wait.

Most days I just vegetated. For months, I traveled from the couch, to the recliner, to the bed. I sensed God's presence intimately during this time of solitude and recovery. I felt too weak to even hold my Bible and lacked the concentration to read. I fought anxiety daily. I was learning a lot about waiting on the Lord; to renew my strength. Everything required WAITING! Sometimes I would sing very softly and pray while lying in bed, or I'd just "veg out."

I recently experienced "waiting-"-on--God--to--renew--my--strength experience once again while on a medical mission trip. Our mission was to do cataract surgeries for the blind in the impoverished country of Indonesia. On our biggest surgical day I became ill before our fourth case and had to leave the O.R. We had fourteen cases scheduled.

Extreme nausea and fatigue crashed over me. I had to find somewhere to lie down. I thought, *Maybe it's the heat. Or jet lag—or both.* All I knew was that if I didn't lie down; I would fall down! I went promptly to my quarters on the mission compound.

After a two hour deep sleep; I awoke, but didn't rise from the bed. My head felt like I was a wearing a diver's bell. My arms felt like heavy weights.

As I lay there, I pondered the morning devotional we shared. Again, it was Isaiah 40:29, "THEY THAT *WAIT* UPON THE LORD, SHALL RENEW THEIR STRENGTH."

Didn't God know I was there to help with crucial surgical cases? I didn't have time to wait! I needed to help! Didn't I?

As I rested there, I began to pray for my team mates who were hard at work. I prayed for my family back home and for the women in my small group. As I continued to wait upon the Lord in my weakness; I envisioned the face of a Chinese man named Chiang Li. We had done surgery on his right eye. I couldn't get his face out of my mind. So, I began praying for him…He was blind in both eyes….His face was downcast; his pupils darted to and fro; searching for the light…..He was in the dark….completely. He was only 35 years old and he'd been blind for over a year already.

(Oh, by the way---you'll have **to wait** for part Two **to see** what happens to Chiang Li.)

GRACE TO WAIT

Hate to Wait -- Part Two

Chiang Li hadn't worked in over a year due to his blindness from dense cataracts. With his hand on his wife's shoulder, he would follow closely behind her. There are no white canes or guide dogs in the jungle villages of Borneo. No social security for his disability. No eye surgeons nearby to perform the surgery that could restore his sight. No money to travel to find one.

That was our mission; to bring sight to the blind. Chiang Li was one of our first surgical cases of the week. He was also diabetic and dependent on insulin; which raised the risk of even more vision loss.

The next day after his surgery, Chiang Li not only looked like a different person; he was looking at everyone and everything! Out of the darkness and into the light! His gaze was often focused on his wife's face; their hands were clenched together tightly as they waited for his post op check. His countenance was completely different now. From hopelessness to gratitude and joy; a smile replaced the prior downcast appearance.

We informed Chiang Li that we would do surgery on his other eye the next week if we had time. We had more bilaterally blind patients to do first.

A person can function very well with vision in one eye. We wanted to help as many as we could in our two week stay.

On our last surgical day there; we had seven cases lined up. We put Chiang Li on as our last case. We ended up having just enough time to give him cataract surgery with intraocular lenses on both eyes. I felt compelled to tell him of God's great love for him and to ask him if it would be alright if we prayed for him. But I didn't speak Indonesian or Chinese! I needed someone who did to translate. And so, I prayed, "Lord, if you want me to speak to this man; you'll have to provide someone to translate."

We finished our third case, then the fourth, then the fifth. Suddenly my answer to prayer walked into the room. It was Jennifer, a missionary nurse who had lived there for the past four years. She spoke the language very well; and had a heart to pray for others!

Three of us went to the room next to the operating room. I began to tell him of God's great love for him--that God sent us specifically to help him regain his sight. He said, "I have no religion."

I asked him if he would allow me to pray for him; just as he allowed us to do surgery on his eyes to remove his blindness. He agreed. I prayed that God would remove the blindness from the eyes of his heart; and that he would come to know that Jesus is the Way, the Truth and the Life.

Chiang Li smiled and said, "Tareema Kasi", which means "Thank you."

I pondered our prayer time with him while on return flight to the U.S.. I was reminded that, in Ephesian's 1: 17 - 18, the apostle Paul writes, "I keep asking that the God of our Lord Jesus Christ, the glorious Father, may give you the Spirit of wisdom and revelation, so that you may know him better. I pray also that the eyes of your heart may be enlightened in order that you may know the hope to which he has called you...."

I also mused about the many patients we saw and for whom we provided surgery; and yet it was only one man I felt compelled to pray for and to tell him about Jesus. I remembered that Jesus is the Good Shepherd. And as a good shepherd does; he leaves the ninety nine to search for the *one* lost sheep.

Though I still hate to wait at times; I now understand that God does his work through the waiting times; and in times of weakness his power is made perfect. Prayer is *the preceeder* of God's power. You may have heard "When we work; we work. But when we pray, God works."

If you are in God's waiting room; perhaps recovering from surgery; between jobs, between being called and being sent; between God's promises and the manifestation of his word to you--be encouraged:.

"THEY THAT WAIT UPON THE LORD, SHALL RENEW THEIR STRENGTH, THEY SHALL MOUNT UP WITH WINGS AS EAGLE²S!" "THEY SHALL RUN AND NOT BE WEARY, THEY SHALL WALK AND NOT FAINT."

P.S.....PRAY WHILE YOU WAIT!!

Grace for Weaning

Giving It Up

A few years ago, my granddaughter had to give her up beloved *binky*. She had her binky ever since she was an infant. She sucked herself to the zone---the comfort zone. The binky and her blanky were all she needed for nap time or nighttime or when she was upset or sick.

I've recently seen some teenagers, even young males, walking around with a binky in their mouths. I'm sure you have seen it too. It is absurd. It looks moronic to me. I don't see what is "*in*" about looking moronic.

Needless to say, I am glad my six--year--old granddaughter does not continue to suck on a binky. She would still be attached to it had her parents not decided she needed to be weaned from it.

One night, soon after soon after she had to *give it up,* I was called upon to baby-sit while her parents went away over-night. I lay down with her to comfort her to sleep. I sang to her, prayed for her, and stroked her silky brown hair in an attempt to help ease the discomfort of her parent's overnight absence for the first time in her little life. Several times I just quietly whispered, "sh, sh, sh".......

I was beginning to feel like a failure as a grandparent. All of my attempts to soothe her appeared to be useless as she flip--flopped like a fish out of water.

She finally cried out, "I want my binky, but daddy won't let me have it!" I felt her pain as I observed her mourning her beloved pacifier.

She was like a junkie without a fix. She was literally going through binky withdrawal. It hurt my heart to see her so distressed. I began to gently rub her back and sing softly. Finally, after much jerking and moaning, she lay still and fell asleep.

We are not much different than small children in distress when our security is taken away from us. What have you become accustomed to as a form of security? It could be your spouse, your job, a parent or a_friend. It could be your savings account or even your own personal appearance or health. But then that thing is suddenly removed. Somehow, our heavenly daddy has seen fit to wean us from some secure person or item in our life and we, too, grieve the loss with tears and moans.

We may or may not toss and turn or flip flop in bed when our "security blanket", is ripped away from us. But even if we are not doing it outwardly, we are often crying out inwardly and our mind is flip flopping with fear and anxiety. Our soul heaves up and down on the ocean of emotion, and feel as though we are sinking in despair.

"Be still, my soul," is what we need to say to ourselves in times of trial. When the rug of comfort has been pulled out from underneath us we need to acknowledge and remember that God has loved us with an everlasting love and underneath are his strong arms of comfort ready to hold us in this life and the life to come.

"Be still and know that I am God." Psalm 46:10. Quiet down that anxious mind and make it to be still. Get in a quiet place and meditate on those words Be still---God is in control. He is not surprised by anything. He knows before you do. Is he not able to quiet the waves on the sea anymore? He spoke to the storm that night when the disciples thought they would perish. When he said to the tempest "Be still," the waves immediately ceased from their roaring.

Like a child who has been weaned, we need to quiet our souls and still ourselves with the comfort of God's promises. It's okay to admit your very human emotions, but, in the end, we must realize fully that our Father knows what is best.

CPSIA information can be obtained
at www.ICGtesting.com
Printed in the USA
FFOW02n1343201015
17844FF